D1710282

Visual Field Defects after Penetrating Missile Wounds of the Brain

Visual Field Defects after Penetrating Missile Wounds of the Brain

HANS-LUKAS TEUBER

WILLIAM S. BATTERSBY

MORRIS B. BENDER

Published

for THE COMMONWEALTH FUND

by HARVARD UNIVERSITY PRESS

Cambridge   1960

Published for The Commonwealth Fund
by Harvard University Press, Cambridge, Massachusetts
Distributed in Great Britain by Oxford University Press, London

For approximately a quarter of a century THE COMMONWEALTH FUND,
through its Division of Publications, sponsored, edited, produced, and
distributed books and pamphlets germane to its purposes and operations
as a philanthropic foundation. On July 1, 1951, the Fund entered into
an arrangement by which HARVARD UNIVERSITY PRESS became the pub-
lisher of Commonwealth Fund books, assuming responsibility for their
production and distribution. The Fund continues to sponsor and edit its
books, and cooperates with the Press in all phases of manufacture and
distribution.

Library of Congress Catalog Card No. 60–8452
Manufactured in the United States of America

For Kurt Goldstein on his eightieth birthday
November 6, 1958

Preface

This monograph tells of observations made by us from time to time over a span of nearly fifteen years. The earliest records go back to the last phase of the second World War when two of us (M. B. B. and H.-L. T.) were stationed at the U.S. Naval Hospital in San Diego, California, from 1943 to 1946. During that period we studied acute effects of penetrating brain injury in Naval casualties of the Pacific campaigns. Three years later this work was resumed at the Psychophysiological Laboratory (New York University–Bellevue Medical Center), a unit devoted primarily to studies of late effects of brain wounds (due to missiles) in a larger group of veterans of the last war. From 1949 to 1952 we had a third collaborator in W. S. Battersby, and many of our initial observations on the veterans' group at the Psychophysiological Laboratory were thus made together. Since 1952 the work has been continued by one of us (H.-L. T.) at the Psychophysiological Laboratory, where this summary was prepared in 1957 and 1958.

In all our studies, whether carried out jointly or separately, our initial concern has been the visual system and its changes with cerebral injury or disease. This emphasis has remained, though supplemented and followed by parallel studies of other sense modalities. The present monograph embodies the original emphasis, being limited to surveys of visual functions as affected by cerebral trauma; other volumes report on changes in somatosensory function after brain injury (Semmes, Weinstein, Ghent, and Teuber, 1960) and on more general effects of this condition on behavior (Teuber, monograph in preparation).

Throughout, our concern has been less with disordered functions as such than with clues they might provide to the physiologic bases of normal func-

tion. Despite certain differences of approach we believe that abnormal function, after brain injury, can and should be studied by methods drawn from
psychophysics and comparative psychology and that such investigations will
bring us closer to an eventual "coalescence of neurology and psychology." It
will be apparent to the reader how much we owe, in this respect, to the three
men who for so long have worked towards the synthesis of neurology and the
study of behavior: Kurt Goldstein, Karl S. Lashley, and Heinrich Klüver. To
the first of these three, we dedicate this monograph on the occasion of his
eightieth birthday.

We are likewise indebted to the institutions and foundations which have
made these protracted studies possible. For the earliest phase of the work, we
owe thanks to the Medical Department of the U.S. Navy, which permitted us
to engage in these investigations at the height of a war and to continue them
into the difficult period of demobilization. The resumption of this work after
the war would have been impossible without the help, both administrative
and financial, of the U.S. Veterans Administration (under Contract V 1001
M-176 with the New York University–Bellevue Medical Center). Further aid
was received from the Office of the Surgeon General (U.S. Army) under Contract
DA-49-007-MD-312 with the Psychophysiological Laboratory. For the last
seven years, however, the entire research program of the Psychophysiological
Laboratory, including the aspects of its work reported in this monograph, was
made possible by the Commonwealth Fund of New York. To the staff of the
Fund, particularly Dr. Charles O. Warren, we are deeply grateful for their
continuous encouragement of our work and their warm, personal support.
Since September 1959, our work continues under a seven-year program grant
(M-3347) from the U.S. Public Health Service (National Institute of Mental
Health).

The monograph in its present form is half text, half pictures. Marianne
L. Teuber drew most of the visual fields, graphs, and diagrams, and arranged
all pictorial material for publication. Louise Pfeiffer, as research secretary of
the Psychophysiological Laboratory, typed and retyped the text, and saw it
through its various revisions. Our debt on both counts cannot be repaid.

A number of friends were kind enough to read part or all of this monograph in its earlier versions and to undertake the thankless task of improving
its exposition. While they cannot be blamed for the shortcomings that remain,
they have helped our readers by helping us. We should mention particularly
Dr. Joseph Altman, Dr. George Ettlinger, Dr. Norman Geschwind, Professor
Pinckney J. Harman, Dr. Jonathan Wegener, Dr. Lawrence Weiskrantz, and
Professor Oliver Zangwill.

H.-L. Teuber

New York, 1960

Table of Contents

1. The Problem

Changes in visual fields after gunshot wounds of the brain have been studied less often than field defects which follow cerebrovascular accidents or space-occupying lesions. Yet most investigators of gunshot wound cases have stressed the importance of such data for understanding the neural basis of visual functions (Holmes and Lister, 1916; Holmes, 1918a,b, 1919a,b; Riddoch, 1917; Poppelreuter, 1917; Spalding, 1952a,b). Field defects after missile wounds tend to be more varied in outline and more stable than those seen in other instances of destruction or irritation in the higher visual pathways. Because of their variety and stability, traumatic cases lend themselves to particularly detailed investigations.

The two main tasks for such a study lie (a) in describing the characteristic features of field defects after missile wounds and (b) in asking to what extent these changes conform to known anatomic arrangements in higher visual pathways. Both tasks are meaningful, despite the lack of autopsies in most traumatic cases.

Mere description of altered visual function can add to our understanding of normal visual physiology, even if site and extent of underlying lesions remain unknown. Different aspects of visual performance are affected in systematically different fashion; some seemingly unrelated functions are disturbed together, while others are readily dissociated. Severe deficits can be

1

compared with those that are slight, and early stages in recovery with later stages, revealing a rank order in the fragility of different aspects of vision, and thus suggesting a hierarchy of functions. The extreme persistence of residual defects after cerebral wounds permits us to observe characteristic patterns of adaptation to these defects, including changes in fixation and space perception, and to contrast this adaptation with that seen in peripheral sensory impairment.

To this end, we made detailed visual field studies of a group of men who had suffered cerebral gunshot wounds many years before testing. Our findings on this group were supplemented by observations on acute visual field changes which we recorded for another group during the first few weeks or months after trauma. All the patients were believed to have been normal before they were wounded. In both instances, we employed a variety of methods in addition to the traditional plotting of visual fields. Among these were flicker perimetry, the measurement of dark adaptation, and assessment of thresholds for perception of real and apparent motion. It was by means of these auxiliary methods that we could determine degrees of impairment in different parts of a field, evaluate the nature of the impairment, and uncover persistent minimal deficits, even in seemingly intact portions of the field of vision. Moreover, the studies provided results bearing on the relative vulnerability of different aspects of normal function.

If all this is possible without autopsies, their absence nevertheless imposes restrictions on attempts at correlating specific deficits in performance with particular lesions in underlying structures. Despite these limitations, studies of field defects after gunshot wounds have made indirect contributions to traditional problems of localization. During the first World War, field defects were noted whose shape supported views on retinocortical projection, based on earlier clinico-pathologic studies (e.g., Niessl von Mayendorf, 1907; Henschen, 1910) and animal experiments (e.g., Minkowski, 1913). Thus, Holmes (1918a, 1919a; Holmes and Lister, 1916; see also Wilbrand and Saenger, 1918) observed field defects in both lower quadrants from bullets traversing the occiput on a horizontal course rostral to a point lying 2 cm. above the occipital protuberance. Defects in the upper quadrants resulted from injuries somewhat below this point. Holmes also recorded instances of blindness restricted to the centers of the visual fields after lesions which involved the tips of the occipital poles. These observations strengthened the belief in a vertical projection (upper half of visual field into lower part of calcarine fissure, and conversely), and supported the view that a similarly simple scheme (an antero-posterior arrangement) might account for representation of concentric zones of the field: the most peripheral zones of the field might be projected most anteriorly, that is, into the depth of the calcarine fissure, and the center of the field most posteriorly, that is, to the occipital pole. Both the vertical and the antero-posterior projection seemed involved in producing the strange field defects illustrated in Figures 1 and 2.

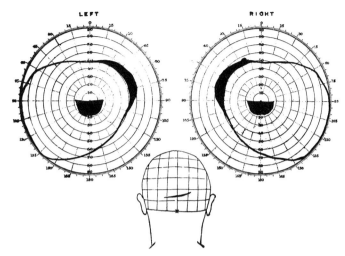

Figure 1. Homonymous field defects recorded by Holmes and Lister for a case of gutter-type gunshot wound impinging on the occiput about 2.5 cm. above the pro-tuberance. Note restriction of the defects to lower homonymous halves of the macular and perimacular areas. Target used: white, 6 mm. in diameter.

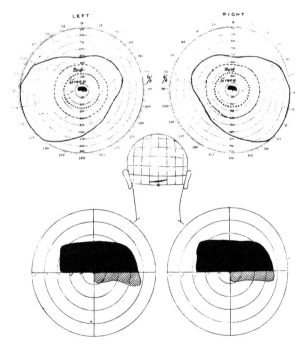

Figure 2. Homonymous field defects recorded by Holmes and Lister for a case of gutter-type gunshot wound traversing the occiput just above the occipital protuber-ance. Note that the defects are in the upper homonymous halves of the macular areas, in a manner roughly complementary to those illustrated in Figure 1. Targets used: white, 7 mm. in diameter; red and green, 10 mm. in diameter.

Both reproduced by permission from G. Holmes, *Brit. J. Ophthal.* 2:353–384(1918).

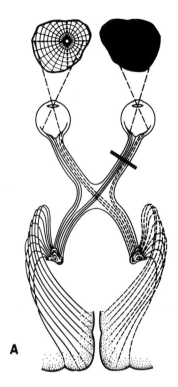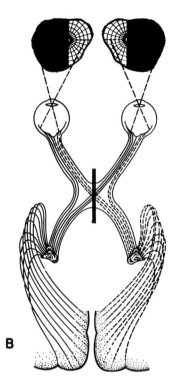

Figure 3. Diagrams of man's visual pathways and visual field defects (black) resulting from lesions in different locations.

A. Monocular blindness (right eye) due to lesion of right optic nerve.

B. Heteronymous hemianopia (in the temporal halves of both fields) due to lesion involving the crossing fibers in the chiasm; note that only the nasal portions of the field are spared. Other lesions of the chiasm may occasionally produce the converse; a binasal hemianopia. Such defects (bitemporal, binasal) are called "heteronymous" (of different name) because one field shows loss in the right half, the other in the left.

C. Homonymous hemianopia involving the left halves of each field (nasal for right eye, temporal for left) due to interruption of either the optic tract on the right or the right optic radiation. All field defects charted in Diagrams C–F are "homonymous," since lesions posterior to the chiasm in the right hemisphere implicate the left halves of each field; correspondingly, retrochiasmal lesions in the left hemisphere implicate the right halves of each field. The exceptions to this statement are the rare instances of selective loss of one monocular crescent (see Figs. 34 and 35).

D. Homonymous defects in left upper quadrants due to partial interruption of right optic radiation, presumably in its ventral (lower) sector.

E. Homonymous defects in left lower quadrants due to partial interruption of right optic radiation, presumably in its dorsal (upper) sector.

F. Homonymous hemianopia involving the left halves of each field due to destruction of terminal projection of optic radiation in the right occipital lobe. See text for further details, particularly the problems of macular sparing.

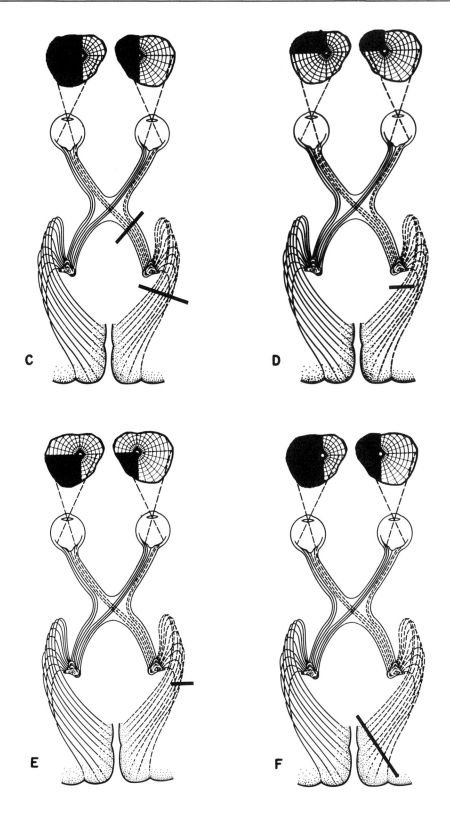

Findings such as these agree with available notions about representation, since the fields tend to corroborate what histologic studies have demonstrated in advance. However, there are other observations of equal or greater importance: those that cannot be predicted by existing conceptions of the visual pathways. Throughout the first World War, temporal and deep parietal wounds were observed to produce quadrantic defects. Holmes (1919a) and, independently, Monbrun (1919) pointed out that these quadrantanopiae could not be understood in terms of then current views on the course of the optic radiations. The pathway from lateral geniculate to striate cortex was known to be a single bundle; macular fibers (i.e., those representing foveal and perifoveal regions) were thought to be concentrated on the upper or lower margins of the bundle or intermingled with fibers representing the peripheral field.

Holmes as well as Monbrun stressed that the frequent occurrence of defects limited to a peripheral quadrant required the existence of some anatomic interval separating representations of upper and lower peripheral quadrants. Neither Holmes nor Monbrun could say with certainty what this interval might be, though Monbrun had postulated that the gap was filled with centrifugal fibers and with fibers devoid of visual function (Monbrun, 1914, 1919). Rønne, however, suggested in 1919 that the interval was formed by macular fibers interposed between upper and lower parts of the radiation. Over a decade later, Polyak (1932, 1933, 1957) provided histologic evidence for such an arrangement in the optic radiation of the monkey. Polyak (1957) believed that the same arrangement might also be found in man, and his views have been accepted for both species. As we shall see, however, the situation in man is far from clear; quadrantic defects appear in many forms, and some of these cannot be explained in Polyak's terms, particularly with respect to the intermediate course of man's optic radiation.

The field defects we shall describe likewise exhibit both types of features: those that are obviously compatible with current concepts of visual anatomy (Fig. 3) and those that are not. It is the latter type of finding that has potential anatomic significance. If these findings do not answer anatomic questions, they can at least set problems to which future histologic study must address itself. For this reason, we shall give equal emphasis to expected and unexpected features of the field defects we have observed.

2. Cases Studied

The cases studied were drawn from two groups: one consisting primarily of patients tested long after trauma (group A); the other, of patients tested soon after the brain wound was incurred (group SD).

GROUP A

Visual field and visual performance were recorded for 46 men with visual field defects resulting from penetrating gunshot wounds of the brain. In no case was the injury less than five years old at the time of study; the condition was followed, in all but 3 instances, until at least ten years had elapsed after the lesion had been sustained. Of the 46 patients with field defects, 42 had been injured in World War II, 3 in the Korean campaign (designated as AK), and 1 in World War I. All were drawn from a larger series of veterans with battle wounds of the brain, who had been under observation since 1949 (except for those injured in Korea, who entered the program in 1952 and 1953). The total group comprised 232 men, but as the visual fields were plotted in only 206 cases, the 46 patients with field defects represented an incidence of 22 per cent.

This proportion is similar to that reported by other investigators (e.g., Spalding, 1952a; see also Symonds, 1945; McGavic, 1947; and, for reviews,

Duke-Elder, 1949). The comparative rarity of field defects may reflect differences in chances of survival after missile wounds to different parts of the brain. Men with injuries in anterior portions of the cerebrum are apparently more likely to survive than those with involvement of posterior-lobe substance.

GROUP SD

The data obtained from group A (46 veterans) were supplemented by observations made earlier (during World War II at the San Diego Naval Hospital) on Naval casualties, whose visual functions were studied less than one year after they had incurred gunshot wounds of the brain. Composition of groups A and SD otherwise appears identical in all important respects. Systematic descriptions in the present report are limited to group A, the group with injuries of long standing. Cases from group SD are adduced for purposes of additional illustration, and for comparing early and late effects of trauma to the visual pathways.

3. Methods

All 46 patients with permanent field change (group A) were studied over periods extending from several months to eight years.

ROUTINE PERIMETRY

Routine perimetry was performed separately for each eye in a Brombach perimeter, with 1° white targets 330 mm. distant from the cornea, under 7 foot-candles illumination by a daylight bulb. We defined as an absolute scotoma any area in which a patient, under these conditions of testing, was unable to discriminate presence from absence of the 1° white target, as long as the target was held stationary. Such areas are charted throughout in solid black. By contrast, stippled areas on our perimetric charts are intended to show regions of "amblyopia," defined as those regions in which the patient was able to perceive a moving 1° white target but unable to discriminate between its presence and absence soon (10 sec. or less) after the target became stationary (see Riddoch, 1917; Cibis, 1947, 1948; Cibis and Müller, 1948; Bay, 1950, 1953). Each monocular field was plotted while the patient maintained direct forward gaze; however, the nasal border of each field was replotted after the patient's head had been rotated to the opposite side, so that encroachment on the field by the ridge of the nose was minimized. In tests requiring reasonably steady fixation, we placed a luminous circular patch of 1° diameter over the area of the field into which the normal blind spot projected. (This maneuver could not be applied when the blind spot was involved in areas of scotoma or amblyopia.) The patient was instructed to tell the examiner whenever the circular patch came into his view. The examiner would then conclude that the patient's gaze had shifted. This method of controlling fixation, while indirect and subjective, was found particularly helpful in cases of abnormal fixation (see section on pseudo-fovea). The method has been used extensively in our laboratory for perimetry and flicker perimetry in cases of squint (Feinberg, 1956).

CENTRAL FIELDS

Central fields were studied with the campimetric attachments to the same perimeter, under the same illumination. A plane surface was placed inside the perimeter arc and so aligned that the surface was in the patient's frontal plane. The center of the surface was 330 mm. distant from the patient's cornea; as in perimetry, testing was done separately for each eye. The surface on which the fields were charted was rectangular, subtending 20° above and 20° below its center (which served as fixation point), and 25° to the right and left of it. Targets used for plotting the central fields with this campimetric arrangement were ½° white, red, and green pigmented discs. Areas of scotoma and amblyopia were defined and charted as before. It should be pointed out that the campimetric method differs in one obvious respect from perimetry. In the latter a target subtends the same visual angle no matter where it is placed within the arc of the apparatus which forms, in effect, a half-sphere in front of the patient, with the patient's eye at the center of the sphere. In campimetry the targets appear on a flat surface. Thus, they subtend increasingly smaller visual angles as they are moved from the center towards the periphery of the field.

CHECKS ON RELIABILITY

Perimetry and campimetry are methods which depend on the patient's subjective report; for this reason, they are often considered to have little reliability. In neoplastic disease of the brain, or after recent vascular accidents, performance on field tests can be influenced by abnormal fatigability or limited comprehension of the task. In cases of long-standing cerebral injuries due to missiles such factors play a much smaller role, but visual stimuli need to be controlled in order to obtain reproducible results.

In the studies reported here visual fields were taken at least twice, and at different times for each patient. The testing sessions were divided by intervals varying from several weeks in some cases to several years (up to five) in most. In all but 3 cases the fields were retaken by a different examiner, without

reference to charts obtained at earlier dates. Under these conditions, varia-
tions in the fields from one plotting to another did not exceed 2° in the central parts of the field (i.e., the parts within 5° of the fixation point) and
remained below 5° for the peripheral regions. We are therefore convinced
that the repeat-reliability of these methods is sufficient to warrant their use in
the assessment of permanent field defects.

ADJUNCT STUDIES

Flicker Perimetry

The principal adjunct method was flicker perimetry, performed in a
modified Brombach perimeter (see Teuber and Bender, 1948a,b, 1949; Battersby, 1951): the usual targets were replaced by a small front-surface mirror,
movable on the perimeter arc. The mirror reflected light of a gas-discharge
tube (Sylvania R-1130B) which was electronically controlled (Fig. 4). The
light of the tube could be made to flicker at any rate between 1 flash per sec.
and 70 flashes per sec. Light-dark ratio and size of flickering patch could also
be controlled. The patient, instead of reporting the presence or absence of
a target, judged the appearance of the flickering patch (as "flickering" or
"steady"). To avoid difficulties resulting from prolonged inspection of the
flickering light, the patient made each observation by actuating a microswitch
which exposed the test light for 1 sec. In any given position of the patch within
the field of vision, the flash rate was raised gradually by the examiner (from
2 cycles per sec.), until the patient judged the light as steady. The rate was
increased further (by 10 cycles per sec.), and then reduced until the patient
reported flicker. The critical flicker frequency (CFF) for that position in the
field was defined as the arithmetic mean of 6 consecutive threshold determi-
nations, consisting of alternating ascending and descending trials. The light-
dark ratio was held constant at 1. Target sizes were 2° and ½° of arc, and the
luminous output of the tube (presented in a totally dark cabin) was kept at
8.92 apparent foot-candles per foot-square. CFF values were obtained in this
fashion, separately for each eye, for the fovea, and at 15°, 30°, and 45° towards the nasal and temporal sides along the horizontal meridians. The
resulting values, entered upon a plot of the patient's visual field, yielded the
retinal distribution of flicker fusion thresholds.

Other Adjunct Studies

In addition to flicker perimetry, tests were performed to evaluate the
patient's central acuity, color vision, dark adaptation, depth perception, perception of tachistoscopically presented forms, recognition of hidden figures,
and perception of apparent and real motion (results of some of these adjunct
studies have been published elsewhere, e.g., Bender and Teuber, 1947b, 1948;
Krieger and Bender, 1949, 1951; Teuber and Bender, 1948c, 1949, 1950;
Teuber, Battersby, and Bender, 1951; Teuber and Weinstein, 1956).

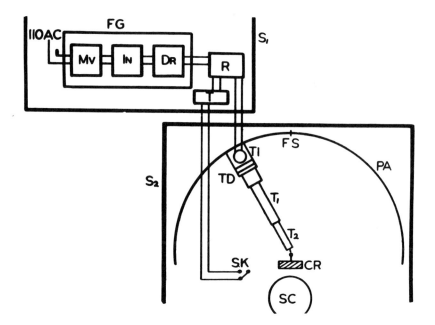

Figure 4. Apparatus employed in flicker perimetry. In the upper left-hand corner, block diagram of flicker generator (FG), surrounded by opaque screen (S₁). The flicker generator consists of a multivibrator (Mv), integrator (In), and driving unit (Dr). The output of this flicker generator is led through appropriate relays (R) which are controlled by an electronic timing unit (T) into the flickering light source placed at TI in the perimeter arc (PA). The perimeter itself is enclosed by another large opaque screen (S₂) which shields the subject's chair (SC) and chin rest (CR). The subject fixates a spot provided by a lucite rod at FS within the perimeter. The output of the flickering source is led through telescopic tubing (T₁, T₂) to the subject's eye. At TD various diaphragms and neutral density filters can be inserted to control size and intensity of the target. The subject makes his judgments by releasing his key at SK which actuates the timing unit and exposes the flickering light for a pre-set duration, usually 1 sec. Flash rate and light-dark ratio are controlled by the experimenter seated behind the flicker generator. For further explanation, see text.

Reproduced by permission from W. S. Battersby, *J. exp. Psychol.* 42:59–68 (1951).

Furthermore, the eye grounds were inspected on at least two separate occasions and always by two different observers. The status of the oculomotor system was also assessed in the usual fashion by testing for adequacy of pupillary response to light, accommodation and convergence; by evaluating pursuit, voluntary shifts of gaze, and involuntary eye movements (nystagmus) upon stimulation by a rotating striped drum.

4. General Composition of the Series

As a group, the 46 patients who were intensively studied after World War II are quite similar to other groups of cases described before and during the first World War (Inouye, 1909; Marie and Chatelin, 1915, 1916a,b; Holmes and Lister, 1916; Riddoch, 1917; Poppelreuter, 1917; Best, 1917, 1919, 1920; Holmes, 1918a,b; Szily, 1918; Wilbrand and Saenger, 1918; Moreau, 1918; Morax, Moreau, and Castelain, 1919; Monbrun, 1919; Gelb and Goldstein, 1920; Uhthoff, 1922; Lenz, 1924; Kleist, 1934).

Judged on the basis of standard perimetry, obvious bilateral involvement of the visual field (19 cases) was found slightly less often than unilateral involvement (27 cases). The upper field was selectively involved in 3 cases, the lower in 4, and the remaining 39 showed involvement in both upper and lower fields. Defects limited to a single quadrant were found in only 7 cases; in 23, two quadrants were involved; in 7, three; and in 9, all four. Some form of hemianopia or hemiamblyopia existed in 18 cases (in 8 the homonymous left halves of the field were involved, in 10 the right homonymous halves). Among these, altitudinal hemianopiae were present in only 3 cases, and in one of these the defect was macular and perimacular. These altitudinal defects were all in the inferior halves of the field.

Quadrantic defects (7 cases) tended to be either smaller or larger than an actual quadrant (see below). In 7 additional cases, the defect consisted of one or several small sector-scotomata. Larger islands of acquired blindness existed in 3 cases. Irregular involvement of three quadrants (usually both lower and one upper) was found in 7 cases. Finally, 3 patients showed marked and irregular contractions, implicating all quadrants of the field, to varying extents. In addition, characteristic arc-shaped defects were noted in 5 cases, always in combination with other forms of scotoma. These arcs or partial rings will be discussed below.

The missiles producing the injuries were shell fragments in 39, and small-caliber projectiles in 7 instances; it may be that the field defects of these 7 patients tended to be somewhat more irregular in outline than those of the others in group A. However, the limited number of cases with wounds from small-caliber weapons does not permit generalization.

The wound of entrance (and site of retained foreign bodies, if any) was charted on standard diagrams of the skull. By means of transparent templates, the location of the penetrating wound was then classified, as involving the right or left hemisphere, or both, and as involving any one or several of the various cerebral lobes. According to this classification of the 46 cases with field defects, the injury was in the occipital region in 11 cases, in the parieto-occipital in 14, and in the parieto-temporo-occipital in 6. In 2 cases all lobes (frontal, temporal, parietal, occipital) were involved. The remaining 13 cases were distributed as follows: 4 fronto-parieto-temporal, 4 parieto-temporal, 2 bilateral parietal, and 1 each fronto-parietal, temporal, and parietal.

These classifications must remain tentative as long as autopsies are lacking, but for the most part errors of localization introduced by our methods underestimate the extent of intracranial destruction. By the same token, the sites of the entrance wounds, and the minimal extent of these wounds, are probably represented with sufficient accuracy to permit comparisons among contrasting groups. Hence we have compared "all men with known frontal penetration" with "all men with known penetration of the posterior third of the cranium." It should be noted, in this context, that no field defects were found among cases classified as "frontal." Theoretically, some field defects in groups A and SD might have been produced by lesions of chiasm or optic tracts, but survival after injury to these structures (by penetrating missiles) is unlikely. For this reason, most, if not all, of the field defects described in the present monograph reflect lesions of the suprageniculate pathways.

In nearly all cases, the eye grounds were normal throughout our period of observation. The exceptions to this statement are noted in the individual instances where fundoscopic abnormalities were observed.

5. Shape of Field Defects:
Expected Features

   In describing the field defects we have observed, we shall begin with features that are readily explained in terms of known arrangements in central visual pathways. From these features, we turn to others that might require certain revisions of current anatomic views. Still later, in Chapters 6 and 7, we shall deal with aspects of vision in a defective field that have little relation to what is known of visual anatomy and physiology.
   In the present chapter we shall consider, in order, four aspects of retinotopical projection, or the way in which visual field and retina seem to be mapped, area for area, into optic radiation and striate cortex: We start with those field defects that are restricted to regions below or above the horizonal meridian of the field. Such altitudinal defects illustrate the principle of vertical projection, whereby upper parts of the field are mapped into the lower portions of the radiation and striate cortex, and the lower parts of the field into the upper.
   After that, we shall describe field defects restricted to the central portions of the visual field. Such defects require discussion of a principle of anteroposterior projection: Since the retina is concave within the eye, one can say that the area of fixation is most posterior, with the zones corresponding to more peripheral areas of the field increasingly anterior, towards the anterior margins of the retina. Field defects that involve, selectively, the central parts

of the field might be understood by making a similar assumption about the arrangement in the striate cortex: The most posterior part of the striate, at the lips of the calcarine fissure, might represent the central parts of the visual field, and the more anterior parts of the striate, in the depth of the calcarine fissure, might represent increasingly peripheral regions of retina and visual field.

Next, we shall try to show that the same arrangement might account for the projection of concentric zones of retina and field into the striate cortex, e.g., for the occurrence of concentrically contracted fields or certain forms of ring-shaped and arc-shaped scotoma.

Finally, we shall turn to a discussion of quadrantic field defects and their relation to some possible disposition of neural elements in optic radiation and cortex. As will become apparent, the anatomic interpretations, inferential from the start, will become increasingly tentative, as we move from a discussion of altitudinal defects to those involving the central parts of the field, and from these to concentric contraction, and to the various forms that quadrant defects can take.

The Principle of Vertical Projection

Inferior Altitudinal Defects

Confirming Holmes' reports (1918a, 1919a), we found that gutter-type wounds produced by missiles passing horizontally along the occiput tend to result in field defects in both lower quadrants, when the path of the missile is somewhat above the tips of the occipital lobes. Such "inferior altitudinal hemianopiae" may be complete, that is, obliterate both lower quadrants, as in case A-71 (see Fig. 5) and case A-140, or may be limited to macular and perimacular regions, as in case A-102 (see Figs. 6a,b). Two of these cases showed a slight and irregular involvement of one upper quadrant, in addition to the bilateral implication of the lower field. It is of interest to note that monocular diplopia (see below, p. 105) developed in two cases: chronic in one (A-102), and intermittent in the other (A-140).

Superior Altitudinal Defects

If the tangential path of the missile lies somewhat below the tips of the occipital poles (cf. Holmes and Lister, 1916), both upper quadrants of the visual field tend to become involved, so that the patient acquires a superior altitudinal hemianopia. No case in our series showed such defects, although there were three (A-71, A-102, and A-140, cited above), whose fields approximated inferior altitudinal hemianopiae.

Earlier studies have stressed that superior altitudinal defects are extremely rare after gunshot wounds (e.g., Marie and Chatelin, 1915; Holmes and Lister, 1916; Best, 1917; Lenz, 1924). The rarity of superior defects is probably related to the proximity of the lower bank of the calcarine fissure to venous sinuses, and to vital structures in the brainstem. Absence of altitudinal hemianopiae in the upper fields thus does not detract from the established views on vertical

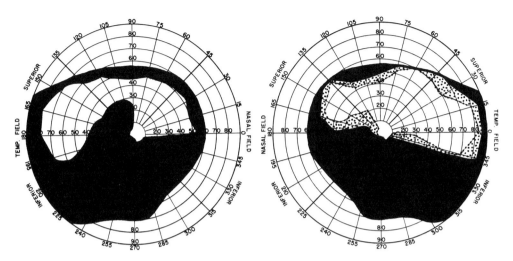

Figure 5. Case A-71. Irregular altitudinal hemianopia in the inferior halves of the fields, due to penetrating gunshot wound (rifle bullet) traversing the occipital region horizontally, 3 cm. above the occipital protuberance. In these and all subsequent visual field charts, the field for the left eye (OS) appears on the left, and that for the right eye (OD), on the right.

projection which ascribe representation of the upper half of the visual field to the lower bank and lip of the calcarine fissure, and the lower half of the field to its upper portions.

THE PRINCIPLE OF ANTERO-POSTERIOR PROJECTION

Macular Defects

Persistent selective involvement of central areas of the visual fields is a surprisingly frequent result of lesions penetrating the posterior brain substance (see our cases A-66, A-76, A-89, A-109, and A-124). Such defects are usually called "macular," although, as Spalding points out (1952a,b), the extent of the macula varies somewhat unpredictably from author to author and is rarely defined. For our present purposes, one can accept the definition by Putnam and Liebman (1942), who propose that the macula be considered to subtend 9° of arc, and the fovea centralis 2°.

Complete loss of macular vision, thus defined, has been reported earlier by one of us, M.B.B. (Bender and Furlow, 1945a,b; see case SD-B, Figs. 7a–c). These central scotomata, which eliminate macular and perimacular vision with preservation of the periphery, are probably due to destruction of the tips of the occipital poles, as in case SD-B (see x-ray of skull, Fig. 7b). Such an observation is thus compatible with Holmes' view on antero-posterior representation which places the macular representation at the most posterior part of the visual cortex, that is, the upper and lower lips of the calcarine fissure, and assigns the more anterior portions, in the depth of the fissure, to the periphery of the field.

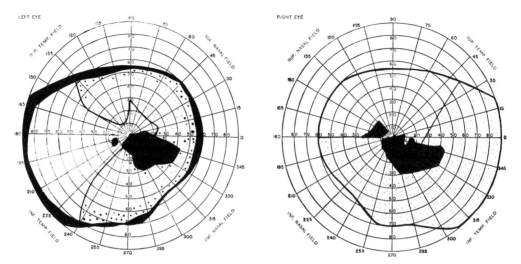

Figure 6a. Case A-102. Irregular and incomplete inferior hemianopia, homony-mous, from penetrating occipital wound, combined with a monocular scotoma in the upper nasal quadrant of the right eye, caused by coincident rupture of the chorioid. A retinal scar, corresponding in location to this monocular scotoma, could be visualized in the right eye on fundoscopy. Note the irregular areas of amblyopia and fluctuation of thresholds, indicated by stippling. Also note the downward displacement of the normal blind spots, indicative of the formation of a pseudo-fovea. This patient showed monocular diplopia in each eye, with recurrent exacerbations as described on pp. 105–106. Snellen acuity: OS 20/200, OD 20/200, not corrected by lenses.

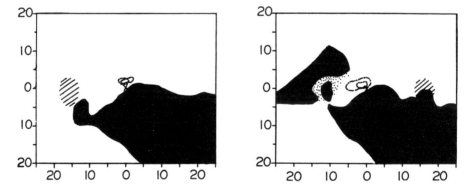

Figure 6b. Campimetric fields obtained for case A-102. Note again the marked downward displacement of the normal blind spots from their expected location in the fields; this suggests that the patient habitually lowered his gaze to minimize encroachment of his homonymous scotomata on visual objects appearing in the central fields. Note also the minute diameter of the fields for color (fields for ½° green surrounded by fields for ½° red).

Wedge-shaped Scotomata

More frequent than total loss of macular vision are instances of incomplete defects involving macular and perimacular quadrants. These defects often assume a characteristic wedge-shape pointing toward the fovea (small sector-scotomata) (see case A-66, Fig. 8; and also Spalding, 1952a,b). Occasionally, such wedges appear at some distance from the center of the field, as in case SD-Mc (Fig. 9). The extreme instance of multiple sector-defects is represented by one of our patients, who exhibited one small homonymous scotoma in each of his macular quadrants, a butterfly-shaped macular field defect (case A-76, Figs. 10a–d).

It is particularly remarkable that this patient insisted for years on working in a travel agency, where he had to look up train and plane schedules in spite of the cluster of scotomata which obstructed his central visual field. He experienced only moderate difficulties in reading and comprehension but made frequent errors in the use of time tables by straying into the wrong line on the page. He finally changed his job to that of interpreter at an international airport, where he could use his equal command of English and Spanish but did not have to do as much reading as before.

The principle of antero-posterior projection suggests that partial defects of macular vision could be caused by partial destruction at the occipital poles. However, it is not immediately apparent why such partial macular defects should be predominately wedge-shaped, nor is it clear that such wedges, or sector-scotomata, should always be attributable to cortical lesions (e.g., as claimed by Polyak, 1957).

In most instances of sector-scotoma, the wedges taper toward the center of the visual fields, so that the pointed ends are near or in the fovea, the broad ends in the periphery. These scotomata may reflect a more extensive representation of the macula, as against the periphery, in the temporal and occipital lobes. On this assumption, a missile which penetrates the posterior lobe substance, and produces an area of destruction of equal width throughout the radiation or calcarine cortex, may leave defects which appear more extensive in the periphery of the fields, an area whose cerebral representation is relatively compressed. This interpretation conforms to electrophysiologic maps of the visual cortex in monkey and cat (see Marshall and Talbot, 1942), but finds less support in actual cell and fiber counts for the central visual pathway, which so far show little of the supposed magnification of the central core representing the macula (see Chow, Blum, and Blum, 1950).

Even less certain is the presumed cortical origin of all sector defects or of sector-shaped rests, i.e., selective involvement or selective sparing of sector-shaped macular regions. Polyak (1957) advanced this postulate primarily for a negative reason: in the cross section of the optic radiation, according to him, macular fibers are concentrated at an intermediate height, with peripheral fibers segregated above and below (Polyak, 1932, 1933). We shall discuss

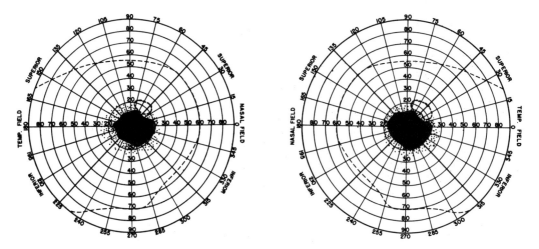

Figure 7a. Case SD-B. Homonymous insular scotomata eliminating macular and perimacular vision in a case of penetrating bullet wound of the occiput. The broken outline above the superior margin of each scotoma indicates an area in which the patient could discriminate among red, blue, and gray targets of 1°. This patient was unaware of the scotomata; he complained merely of a reduction of visual acuity, particularly for objects below his fixation point, which apparently came to lie somewhere at the upper margin of the large central scotomata.

Figure 7b. X-ray of skull (right lateral view), case SD-B. The bullet entered through the right occipital region and made its exit through the left occipital region, leaving two symmetrical wounds, each 2.5 cm. above and 5 cm. lateral to the occipital protuberance. Note indriven bone fragments.

Figure 7c. X-ray of skull (left lateral view) taken during pneumoencephalography, case SD-B. Note again the bullet wounds in the occipital region. There is very slight dilatation of the ventricular system and moderate upward displacement of the right posterior horn. Bone fragments are seen in the brain substance in close apposition to both posterior horns, but none of them appear to have entered the ventricular system. There are trephine holes in the parietal region.

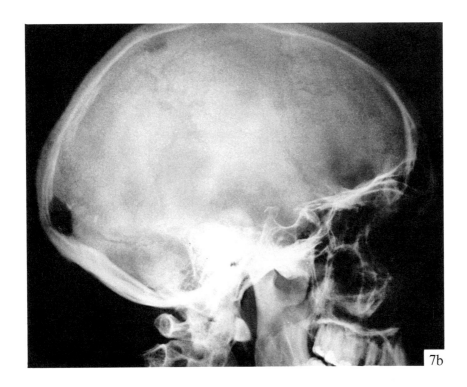

7b

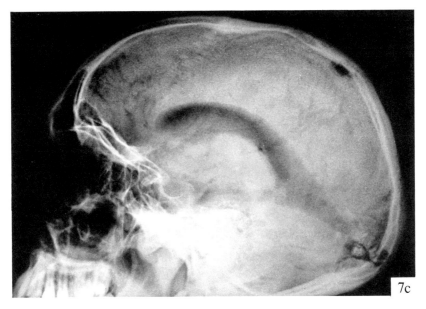

7c

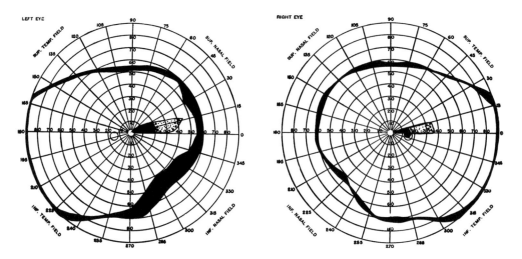

Figure 8. Case A-66. Homonymous sector-scotomata in right superior quadrants tapering towards the fovea. Note the greater extent and density of the scotomata on the nasal side (left eye), as compared with the temporal side (right eye). The field defects were due to a penetrating shell-fragment wound of the left anterior temporal lobe.

Reproduced by permission from H.-L. Teuber, chapter in *Evolution of Nervous Control* (Washington, D. C., AAAS, 1959).

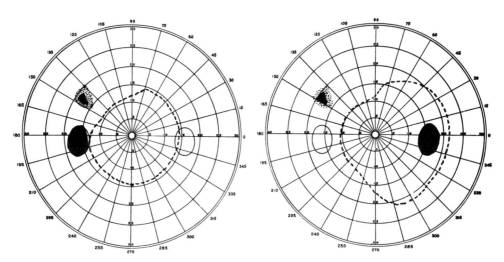

Figure 9. Case SD-Mc. Minute homonymous sector-scotomata in left upper quadrants, tapering towards the fovea. Note that these sector defects, in contrast to the scotomata in 5 other cases, appear to be situated at a considerable distance from the fovea. Also note the contraction in the fields for color (area in which patient discriminated among red, blue, and green 1° targets), in relationship to the position of the small wedge-shaped scotomata in the left upper quadrants.

this proposed arrangement in detail on pages 40–53. If the optic radiation were in fact organized in this manner, wedge-shaped defects like those illustrated in Figure 8 (case A-66) should not result from penetrating wounds of the radiation. The striking wedge-shaped scotomata in this case were produced by a shell fragment entering the left antero-temporal region, from which it was subsequently removed. Remote effects of such a lesion cannot be excluded, but the case makes one hesitate to accept Polyak's view.

On the other hand, most cases of incomplete macular scotoma are probably due to partial destruction at the occipital pole (e.g., cases A-76, Figs. 10a, b; A-89, A-109, A-124), since the wounds of entrance in all these cases were found to be at or near the occipital protuberance, thus implicating what is generally believed to be the foveal projection. A logical extension of this view leads to the idea that concentric zones of the field, surrounding the fovea, should find their representation from back to front, with the most peripheral zones lying most anteriorly, that is, at the depth of the fissure. Such an arrangement suggests the possibility of various "zonal" or arc-shaped defects and of selective losses of the periphery of the field (concentric contraction). In the next section we shall inquire to what extent the defects we have found conform to these predictions.

THE PROJECTION OF CONCENTRIC ZONES

Tubular Fields

Permanently contracted fields result not infrequently from gunshot wounds, especially when the missile passes through the posterior-lobe substance well anterior to the posterior pole (Holmes and Lister, 1916; Wilbrand and Saenger, 1917; see their Fig. 172; Monbrun and Gautrand, 1920). These cases have been counted among the strongest arguments for a topographic arrangement of retinal zones in the calcarine cortex, with the macular regions represented at the posterior pole, and increasingly peripheral zones of the retina represented more anteriorly in the depth of the calcarine fissure.

The situation may be similar in neoplastic involvement of the occipital lobe (cf. Bender and Battersby, 1958), where, early in the disease, one can observe homonymous scotomata in macular or paramacular regions. As the lesion progresses, peripheral parts of the field may become involved, and these peripheral defects grow towards the center and eventually merge with the macular or paramacular scotomata. In temporal or parietal neoplasms, the pattern of progression of field defects with expanding lesions is essentially from peripheral to central parts of the field, and recovery of the field (where it does occur) takes place in reverse sequence, from center to periphery.

In our own series of cases, a permanent bilateral contraction of the peripheral fields can be seen in A-10, A-26 (Figs. 11a,b and 12a,b) and, maximally, in A-29 (Figs. 13a–d). The complementary condition is complete, selective loss of macular and perimacular vision (Figs. 7a,b), with sparing of the periphery.

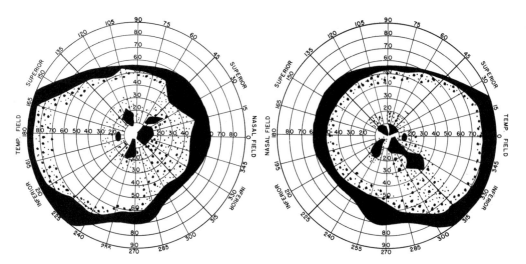

Figure 10a. Case A-76. Multiple sector-scotomata, homonymous, in the perimacular regions, with one major scotoma occupying each of the four quadrants. The field defects were caused by shell fragments which penetrated the occipital bone to the right and left of the midline, from 1.5 to 4 cm. above the protuberance.

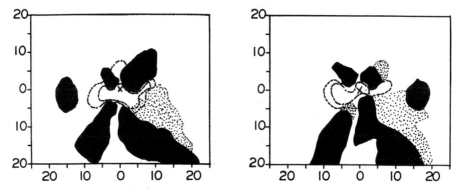

Figure 10b. Central fields obtained for case A-76. Note the lack of congruence of the perimacular scotomata, as well as the irregular outline of the color fields for ½° green targets, surrounded by color fields for ½° red targets.

Figures 10c,d. Left lateral and antero-posterior views of x-ray of skull, case A-76. Note that the occipital bone defect has been extended to the left of the midline during surgery for removal of multiple shell fragments. A single dural clip is seen lying in the occipital region, approximately in midline.

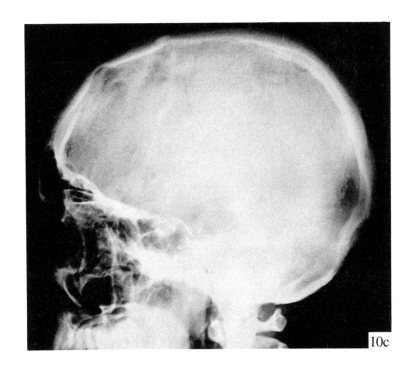

10c

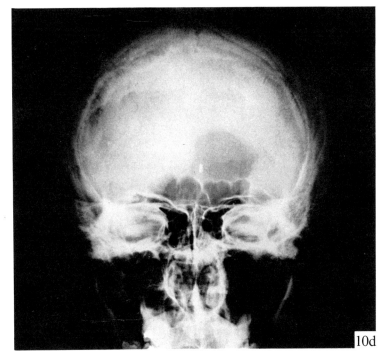

10d

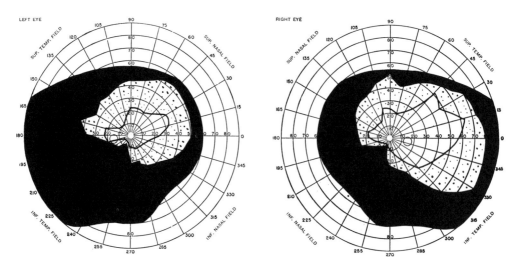

Figure 11a. Case A-10. Homonymous field defects primarily in three quadrants (left upper and lower, right lower) resulting in an irregularly contracted field of vision.

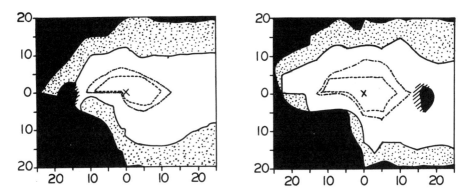

Figure 11b. Central fields obtained for case A-10. Note again how fields for color (½° green surrounded by ½° red) approximately duplicate the contours of the (much wider) fields for the 1° white target.

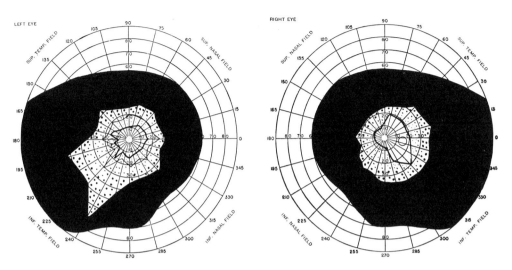

Figure 12a. Case A-26. Concentrically contracted fields with irregular outline taken with 1° white targets. In the stippled region between the solid black area and the ragged line near the 20° isopter, the 1° white target became invisible within 1–2 sec. after it was held stationary. In the central region bounded by the heavy continuous line the patient was able to discriminate presence from absence of the 1° target even when the target was stationary.

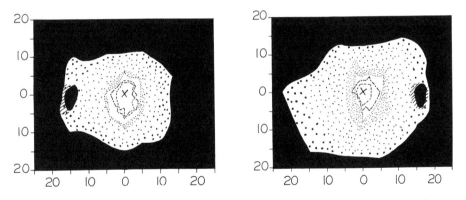

Figure 12b. Concentrically contracted fields, taken on a tangent screen, for case A-26. Since peripheral targets on the tangent screen are at greater distance than central targets (in contrast to targets on the perimeter which maintain their angular size in different retinal positions), this patient exhibited increased contraction of his fields when they were plotted on the tangent screen. Stippling again indicates fluctuation and abnormally rapid disappearance of stationary targets. Note the minimal diameter of the fields for color (field for green surrounded by field for red).

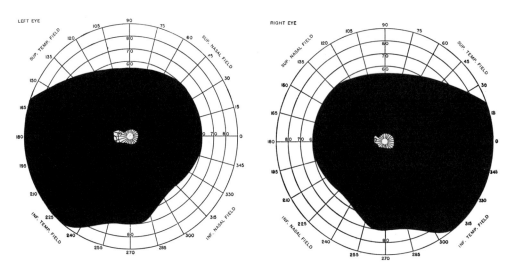

Figure 13a. Case A-29. Extreme instance of concentric contraction, resulting in bilateral hemianopia with irregular macular sparing (peephole vision). Areas in black were blind for hand motion on the perimeter. This unusual type of field defect was the result of a through-and-through bullet wound of the head entering 1 cm. above the pinna of the left ear and making its exit in the right occipital region about 2 cm. above the protuberance and 3 cm. lateral to it.

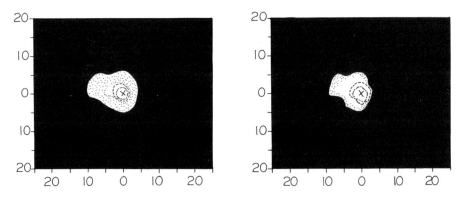

Figure 13b. Central fields obtained for case A-29, showing increased contraction on the tangent screen as compared with the perimetric fields. The fields for color are minute but present. In spite of his peephole vision, the patient had binocular depth perception and essentially normal size and form constancy. By contrast his visual searching behavior was markedly abnormal, showing prolongation of searching times in all quadrants. Fusion thresholds for flickering light were markedly reduced, and dark adaptation was abnormal, as shown in Figure 50. Snellen acuity also was reduced (OS 20/50, OD 20/40).

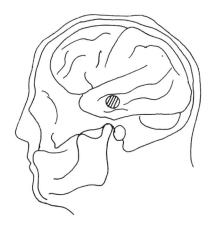

Figures 13c,d. Case A-29. Lateral view (diagram) and postero-anterior view of the skull of the patient, whose fields are illustrated in Figures 13a,b. The wound of entrance, measuring 2.5 x 3 cm., can be seen in the left temporal region. Multiple shell fragments are retained intracerebrally anterior to, and to the left of, the left mastoid region. Another small metallic foreign body lies in the right occipital lobe, 4 cm. to the right of the midline.

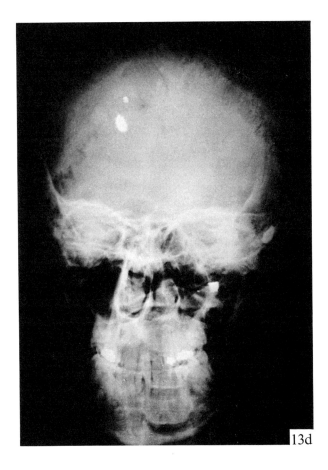

13d

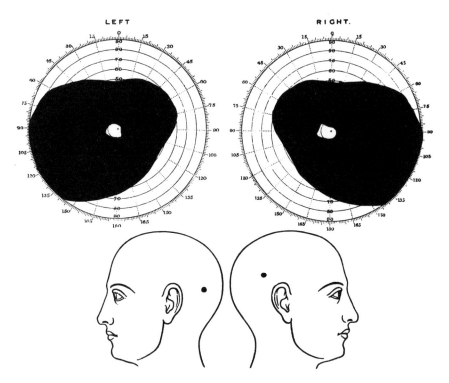

Figure 14. Gordon Holmes' case of bilateral penetration of posterior brain substance, by missile, resulting in bilateral hemianopia with macular sparing. Note the striking similarity with our case A-29 (Fig. 13), including the jagged but homonymous contour of the preserved central field and the oblique curve of the penetrating missile.

Reproduced by permission from G. Holmes and W. T. Lister, *Brain* 39:34–73 (1916).

All 3 cases with concentric contraction had indeed a history of penetration anterior to the occipital pole. However, material of this sort, without anatomic controls, is difficult to interpret.

    If one assumes that concentric contraction, i.e., loss of all peripheral regions of the field is due to destruction of the anterior ends (the depth) of the calcarine fissure, one must explain how the macular fibers in the optic radiations, on their passage posteriorly around the horn of the ventricles, could have escaped. A similar, and equally puzzling case of peephole vision has been published by Gordon Holmes at the end of the first World War (see Fig. 14). Partly because of such difficulties of anatomic interpretation, concentrically contracted fields after gunshot wounds are often dismissed as hysterical. However, careful inspection of such fields reveals features which distinguish them from the usual tubular vision of hysterical origin.

    The two principal distinctive characteristics of contracted fields which are not hysterical are, first, the jagged outline of the field (see cases A-10 and A-26;

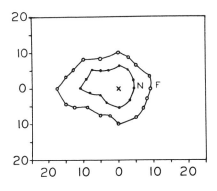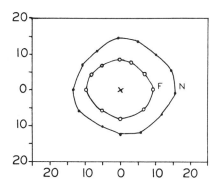

Figure 15. On the left, case A-29: central fields taken for a patient with bilateral hemianopia and peephole vision; the spared parts of the field "widened" as the patient moved farther from the screen. On the right, case A-12: corresponding central fields taken for a patient with right frontal-lobe injury but no demonstrable involvement of the visual structures; the change in the field was paradoxically reversed as the patient moved farther from the screen, indicating that his tunnel vision was of hysterical origin. In each instance the fields were plotted at 1 m. and 2 m. from the tangent screen (N = near, F = far). See text for further details.

Figs. 11a,b and 12a,b) as against the smooth contours of tunnel vision in the hysterical patient; and, secondly, the "widening" of the field with increasing distance. The latter feature provides one with a simple differential test: after plotting the field on a tangent screen, at standard distance, the patient is moved twice as far, the target size is increased correspondingly, and the field replotted. The diameter of the contracted field should now be approximately doubled, as is illustrated for case A-29 in Fig. 15.

In case A-29 the irregular outline of the contracted field was preserved when the field was plotted at twice the standard distance, but the absolute size of the field had increased nearly as much as should be expected according to the law of the visual angle. By contrast, a case of apparently hysterical contraction (case A-12, Fig. 15) yielded a characteristic tunnel field; as the distance between patient and tangent screen was doubled, the field became even more contracted than before—presumably because the patient, unaware of the law of the visual angle, felt that his vision ought to be less efficient at a greater distance. The injury was in the frontal region, with no known involvement of the visual structures.

In making such differential tests, small departures from the law of the visual angle should not be misinterpreted. In several cases of genuine concentric contraction of fields (including A-29), we noted that the field widened with increasing distance, but not quite so much as would be expected on the basis of optic geometry: the patient reacted to the increase in absolute distance of peripheral targets as if his peripheral span were slightly less at greater than at shorter distances. This behavior is reminiscent of that described for normal subjects under the name of Aubert-Foerster phenomenon, but it exceeds in amount what can be demonstrated for normal control subjects, as we have attempted to show in an earlier study (Bender and Teuber, 1947a).

Ring Scotomata

Contracted fields after gunshot wounds seem difficult to reconcile with the usual assumptions regarding the organization of the radiation and cortical retina. This is even more true of annular defects (ring scotomata) and "spiral" defects. As Goldstein has pointed out (1927), it is difficult to accept the view that the corresponding cerebral lesions themselves would have the shape of rings or spirals. Actually, ring scotomata after gunshot wounds are of two kinds: (1) zonal (or arc-shaped) defects, consistent and unvaried from examination to examination, and (2) annular scotomata, varying in position and density from one examination to another.

Arcs. There are permanent defects, such as that seen in case A-67 (Figs. 16a,b), where a half-ring surrounds the macula on the less impaired side, connecting with the amaurotic half of the field above and below the macular region. This defect was consistent from test to test, made by different examiners, over more than two years; it seems to correspond to a lesion involving representations of perimacular zones in upper and lower quadrants on the right.

Defects of this shape should perhaps be designated as "arcs" following Spalding (1952a,b); when incomplete (see Figs. 17a,b; and also Fleischer, 1916, case 2), they have at times been called, picturesquely, "claws" (Brückner, 1917). The incidence of such arcs and claws is rather high after gunshot wounds; they are exemplified by cases 67, 99, 174, 178, and 203 in group A and case C in group SD (see Figs. 16-21). These persistent arc-shaped defects raise serious questions of anatomic interpretation, unless one adopts the views of Holmes (1918a, reaffirmed by Spalding, 1952b), which have already been adduced several times in this report. According to Holmes, concentric arcs of the visual field are represented at successive depths of the calcarine fissure. The arcs closest to the center of the field would be localized in a ring around the entrance of the fissure. Successively more peripheral arcs would then be found at increasing depths of the fissure, with the most peripheral being the most anterior.

It is of course true that the right and left banks of the fissure are in close apposition, so that even small penetrating wounds in the depth of the fissure would easily injure the representations of arc-shaped regions extending across the horizontal as well as the vertical meridians of the field. One has to admit, however, that the situation is likely to be complicated once again by the proximity of deeper parts of the calcarine fissure to the terminal course of the optic radiation.[1] Penetrating lesions involving the depth of the fissure would

---

[1] As a matter of fact, Polyak (1957) categorically attributes arc-shaped defects and remnants (he calls them zonal defects or belts) to lesions of the radiation rather than lesions of the cortex. This assertion, again, would seem to us in need of histologic proof.

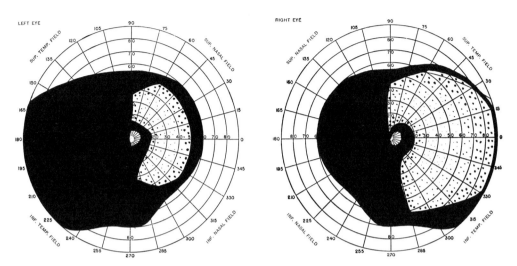

Figure 16a. Case A-67. Left homonymous hemianopia combined with arc-shaped defect forming a half-ring surrounding the right homonymous half of the macular region. This patient was injured by a rifle bullet penetrating the occiput. In the right half-field outside the crescent, fluctuation of targets was marked and stationary targets disappeared within 2–3 sec. Fusion thresholds for flickering light were markedly reduced in the foveal region (i.e., within the arc), and even more so in the right peripheral fields. Apparent movement was reported by this patient when one stationary target was placed inside and another outside the arc-shaped scotoma, and the two targets were illuminated in alternation (see text, pp. 84–86). Snellen acuity: OS 20/100, OD 20/70.

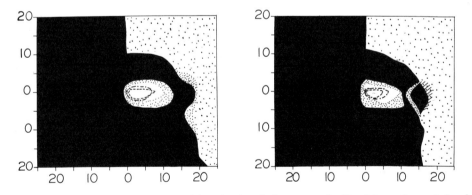

Figure 16b. Tangent screen fields obtained for case A-67. Note the minimal diameter of the color fields within the area surrounded by the arc-shaped scotomata. No color discrimination could be demonstrated beyond the arc, that is, in the periphery of the right homonymous halves of the fields.

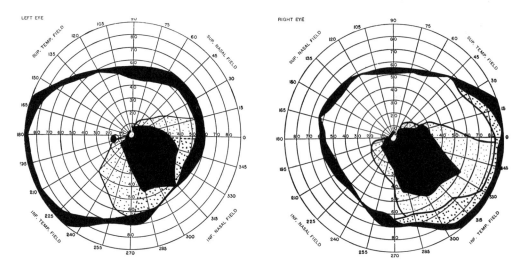

Figure 17a. Case A-99. Large homonymous field defect primarily in the right lower quadrants, combined with an incomplete arc (claw-shaped defect) extending upward around the central portion of the macular field into the left upper quadrants. This field defect was caused by a rifle bullet penetrating the occiput. Snellen acuity: OS 20/20, OD 20/20.

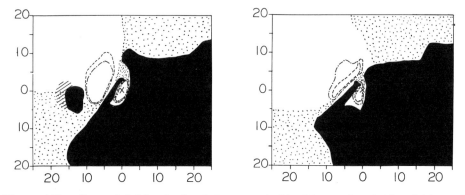

Figure 17b. Central fields obtained for case A-99. Note color fields within and beyond the claw-shaped defect in the left upper quadrants. Also note displacement of the normal blind spot (in the left eye).

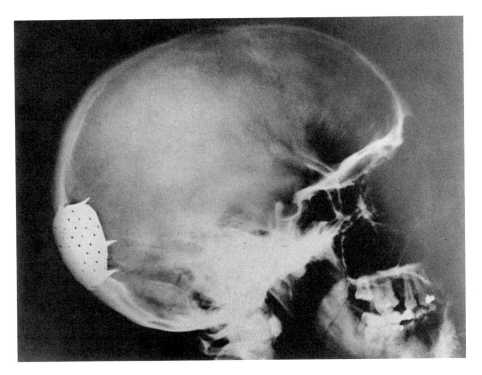

Figure 17c. Right lateral x-ray view of skull, case A–99. A fenestrated tantalum plate covers the occipital bone defect.

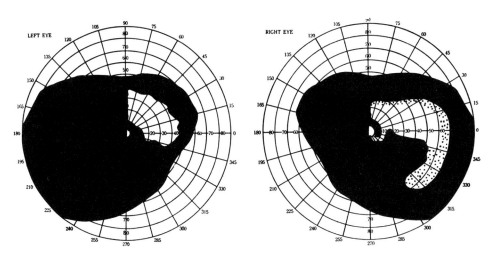

Figure 18. Case A-174. Homonymous field defects in all quadrants, and arc-shaped scotomata in the perimacular right upper quadrants. Note that the arc in the left eye (nasal half) forms a complete half-ring around the spared portion of the macular field, in contrast to the right eye, where the arc is incomplete.

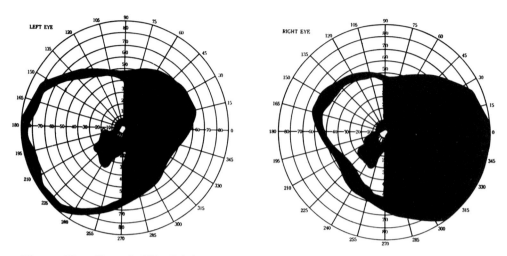

Figure 19a. Case A-178. Right homonymous hemianopia, with irregular defect extending into homonymous left lower quadrants, and arc-shaped defect surrounding the central part of the field. These field defects resulted from a rifle bullet which entered the left midparietal region and traversed the posterior brain substance, making its exit in the right occipital region, 1 cm. to the right of the occipital protuberance.

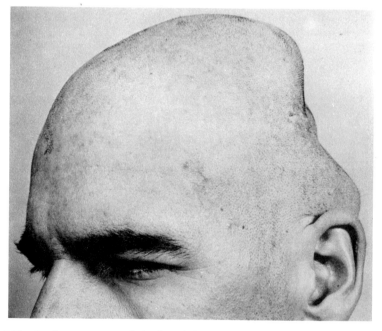

Figures 19b–d. Appearance of the head (case A-178), following surgical removal of fragments from the left midparietal region and the right and left occipital areas.

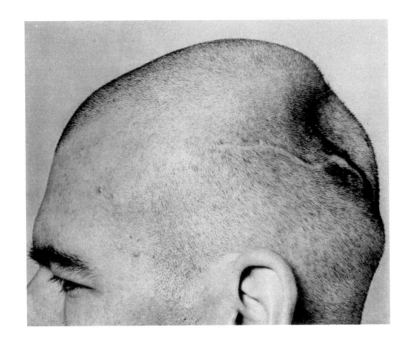

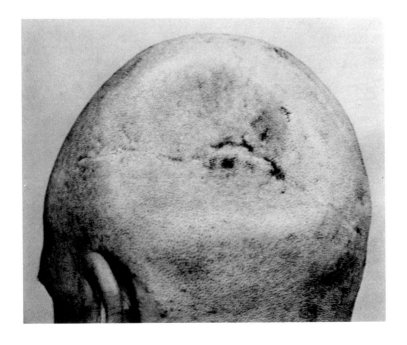

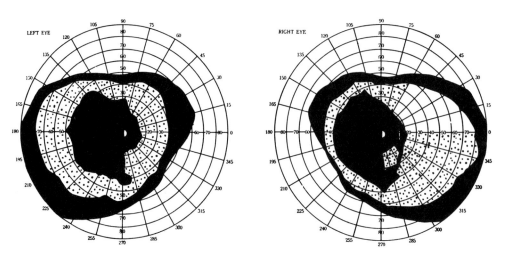

Figure 20. Case A-203. Large irregular homonymous scotomata resulting from penetrating shell-fragment wound of right occipital region, with circular bone defect 2 cm. in diameter. The center of the defect lies 2.5 cm. to the right of the midline and 1.5 cm. above the occipital protuberance. Note the extension of the major scotomata (which are in the left homonymous halves of the fields) into the right half-fields, forming half-rings around minute areas of spared central vision just to the right of the fixation points.

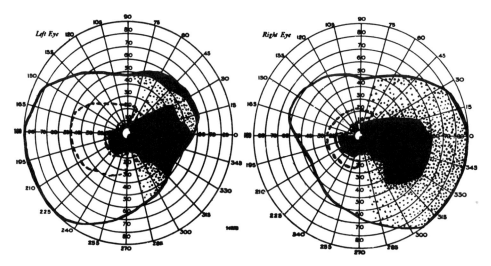

Figure 21. Case SD-C. Irregular homonymous scotomata predominantly in the right half-fields. The patient sustained a penetrating shell-fragment wound in the left occipital region. Three months after injury, his Snellen acuity was 12/15 in each eye. On tests of after-imagery there was marked "completion" of the image through the arc-shaped scotoma on the left; complementary colors were seen in that area.

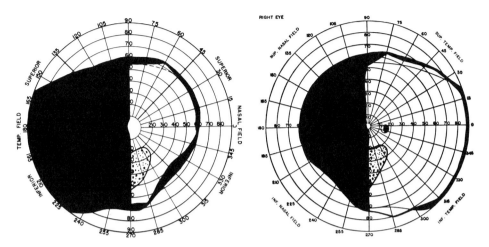

Figure 22a. Case A-82. Left homonymous hemianopia with homonymous ambly-opic defects extending as arc-shaped areas into the right lower quadrants. The field defects were caused by a shell-fragment wound of the right occipital region. When hit, this patient had neither retrograde amnesia nor loss of consciousness; he removed his helmet, noted the hole in it, and realized at the same time that he could not perceive anything to his left. Six days after the wounding numerous bone chips were removed from the right occipital lobe. Post-operatively x-rays revealed a 3.5 x 5.5 cm. bone defect in the right posterior parieto-occipital area, and a small (2 mm.) metallic foreign body lying just within the inner tables of the right occipital region, approximately in line with the lower portion of the bone defect. On repeated testing during the subsequent 12 years, the field defects were found to be unchanged. Snellen acuity: OS 20/25, OD 20/20. Flicker fusion thresholds were depressed in the seemingly intact portions of the fields. No light perception could be demonstrated within the hemianopic regions.

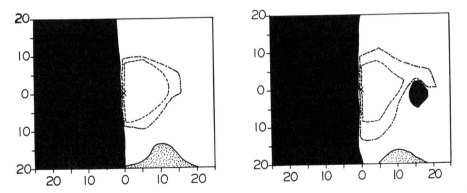

Figure 22b. Campimetric fields obtained for case A-82. Note that the hemianopia is macula-splitting. The color fields for green (inner curve) and red (outer curve) are of nearly normal extent. The normal blind spots are not displaced from their usual position, that is, there are no pseudo-foveae.

be likely to pass through the posterior radiation before encroaching on striate cortex. Such combined lesions of cortex and radiation might account for the various complex field defects illustrated here (Figs. 16–21, i.e., cases A-67, A-99, A-174, A-178, A-203, and SD-C). One should note in particular the frequent tendency of partial quadrantanopiae, or of hemianopiae, to protrude with an arc or even a complete ring into the opposite half of the field. The more peripheral excrescences, or spurs, found in some otherwise simple hemianopiae, e.g., case A-82 (Figs. 22a,b), might possibly be understood by reference to the same considerations.

Variable annular scotomata. In contrast to such permanent and consistent defects are the transient and variable rings or spirals, found occasionally in diffuse lesions, especially after cerebral concussion (see also Iris, 1956). As pointed out by Goldstein (1942, 1943), these cases are not necessarily hysterical. The scotomata can be shown to be due to increased fluctuation of visual thresholds, especially on prolonged exposure of a stationary target.

If the field is plotted in the usual fashion by moving the target slowly inward from the periphery along selected radii, the target tends to disappear ("local adaptation") and reappear when moved farther inward or outward (see Goldstein and Gelb, 1918; Gelb and Goldstein, 1922). When the areas in which the target has disappeared are connected with each other on the plot, a ring scotoma will result; in fact, multiple rings are frequently obtained in this fashion, or even numerous small islands of impaired vision surrounding the fixation point. As we have tried to demonstrate for a special case of temporo-parietal injury by shrapnel (case Ba in group SD; Bender and Teuber, 1947a), the condition is only a general form of what can be observed in the early stages of nearly all impaired fields after gunshot wound of the cerebrum (see also Bay, 1950, 1953). By the same token, these variable ring scotomata and similar manifestations are not found in group A—the patients who were tested several years after their wounding. Group A characteristically shows arcs and claws, which are as little changed from examination to examination, as are the more usual forms of field defect, the hemianopiae, or quadrantanopiae, with which these zonal defects are so frequently combined.

THE PROJECTION OF PERIPHERAL QUADRANTS

Incidence of Quadrantic Defects

Observation of casualties in the Russo-Japanese War of 1904–05 revealed a fairly large proportion of quadrantanopiae among the field defects resulting from brain injury (see Inouye, 1909). These quadrantic defects tended to occupy the upper quadrants after penetration into the temporal lobe, and the lower quadrants after penetration into the depth of the parietal lobe (see also Monbrun, 1914, 1917; Villaret and Rives, 1915; Holmes, 1918a; Wilbrand and Saenger, 1918; Lenz, 1924). Findings such as these, together with observation of similar symptoms after temporal and parietal neoplasms (Fig. 23), led to the

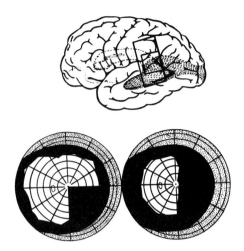

Figure 23. Effects of successive surgical removals from the left hemisphere, presumably involving first only the upper part of the optic radiation and then the entire radiation. Note that the first, smaller resection produced lower quadrant scotomata (probably not as schematic as shown); the larger resection produced hemianopia with macular sparing.

Adapted by permission from J. C. Fox, Jr., and W. J. German, *Arch. Neurol. Psychiat.* 35:808–826 (1936).

schematic view of arrangements within the optic radiation which is still current: in its entire course the optic radiation carries all fibers corresponding to the upper peripheral quadrants of the fields in its ventral portion; fibers corresponding to the lower quadrants are carried in the most rostral portion; interposed between these peripheral representations is the bundle of fibers representing the homonymous halves of the macula (Rønne, 1919; Polyak, 1932, 1933, 1957).

In the standard form of this scheme (the form adopted by current textbooks, e.g., Hughes, 1954), a cross section of the optic radiation (as it courses around the posterior horn of the ventricle) presents itself in the shape of a capital letter C. The uppermost segment of the C contains the lower quadrantic portion of the corresponding (contralateral) monocular crescent. The lowermost segment of the C contains the upper quadrant of the monocular crescent. Above and below these segments one finds the representations of the lower and upper peripheral quadrants, and in the middle of the C, the lower and upper quadrants of the macula (see diagram, Figs. 3 and 29). The question is whether the actual shape of quadrantic defects conforms to this simple scheme.

Incomplete Quadrantanopiae

Strictly quadrantic defects are apparently quite rare after gunshot wounds. In our cases the defects were often partial quadrantanopiae; their characteristic shape was that of a sector-scotoma filling a triangular portion within a quadrant and pointing towards the center of fixation. Such incomplete quadrantanopiae are represented by cases A-182 (Fig. 24) and AK-3; in group SD, case G exhibits a similar phenomenon (Fig. 25).

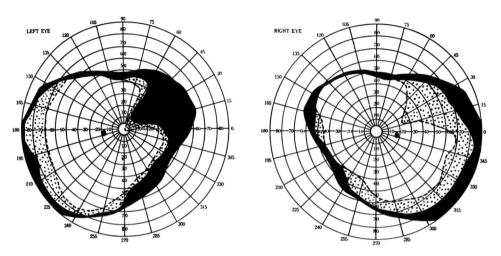

Figure 24. Case A-182. Incomplete quadrantic defects in the homonymous right upper quadrants of the fields. Note that the defect has greater density in the left eye, where it falls into the nasal portion of the field, than in the right eye, where it lies in the temporal part of the field. These defects were caused by a mortar-shell-fragment wound of the left temporal region.

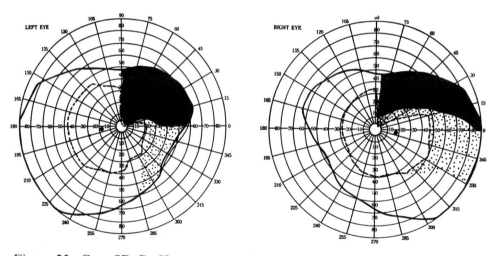

Figure 25. Case SD-G. Homonymous right upper quadrantanopia caused by shell-fragment injury to the left temporal region. Note the lack of congruence of the field defects, due to greater sparing of the horizontal meridian in the right eye. X-rays showed the wound of entrance as a defect of the temporal bone in its most posterior aspect. The defect measured 1 x 2 cm. A large metallic fragment (8 x 13 x 3 mm.) was seen in the midline, in the posterior portion of the skull, 6 cm. from the base and 6.5 cm. from the inner table of the occiput. Several bone fragments were seen in a line extending from the defect in the temporal bone to the site of the metallic foreign body in the depth of the cerebrum.

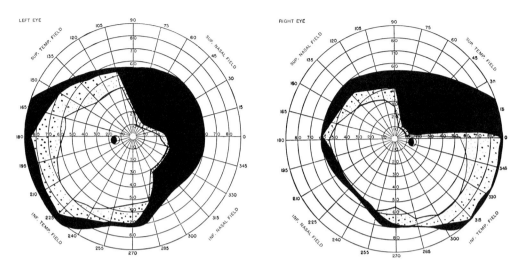

Figure 26. Case A-13. Irregular but homonymous quadrantanopia, with marked overshooting of the defect in the nasal half-field (left eye) into the right lower quadrant. These field defects resulted from a through-and-through wound, caused by a rifle bullet entering the skull in the left frontal region and making its exit in the left temporal region. The patient shows some chorioretinitis of the left eye, where Snellen acuity is 20/200 (acuity in right eye, 20/20).

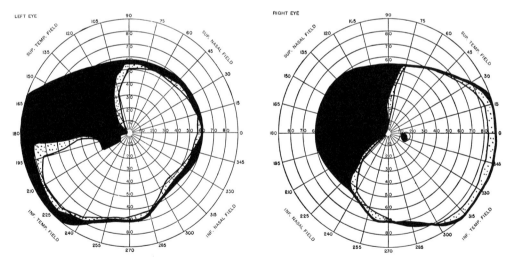

Figure 27. Case A-98. Irregular but homonymous left upper quadrantanopia with overshooting of defect in the nasal half-field (right eye), involving half of the lower left quadrant. The wound of entrance was in the right parieto-temporal region. X-rays showed bone fragments scattered along a line from the skull defect (1 cm. in diam.) to a point just posterior to the sella turcica about 1 cm. to the right of the midline, where a 1.5 x 1.5 cm. foreign body was retained. Pneumo-encephalographic studies showed slight dilatation of the right lateral ventricle; this ventricle was pulled slightly towards the skull defect. Snellen acuity: OS 20/40, OD 20/25.

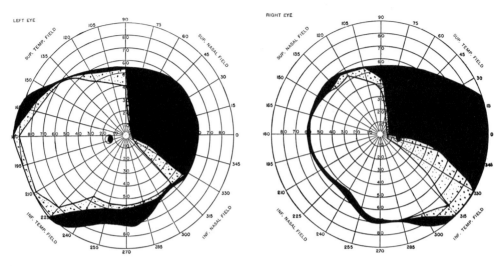

Figure 28a. Case A-30. Right upper quadrantanopia with marked overshooting into the lower quadrants of the fields. A penetrating bomb fragment (3 x 3 mm.) entered through the left supraorbital ridge, traversed most of the left hemisphere, and remained embedded in the depth of the brain, in the left anterior occipital region, just lateral to midline. The dark-adaptation curves obtained for the center of the field and for a point 20° from the fovea in the left upper quadrant were grossly abnormal, as were fusion thresholds for flickering light in the seemingly spared portions of the field. No light perception could be demonstrated in the apparently blind areas of the right upper quadrants. Snellen acuity: OS 20/50, OD 20/40.

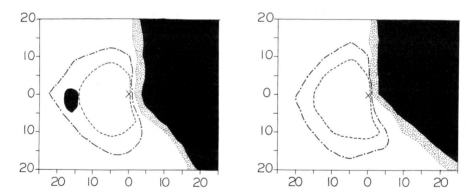

Figure 28b. Campimetric fields obtained for case A-30. Note nearly normal outlines for fields for color in the left half-field, and marked contraction in the right lower quadrants, that is, in the quadrants which (according to standard perimetry, with 1° white targets) appeared to be spared.

Figures 28c,d. X-rays of skull (case A-30) showing foreign body which entered through the left supraorbital ridge, traversed the brain, and lodged in the left posterior lobe substance.

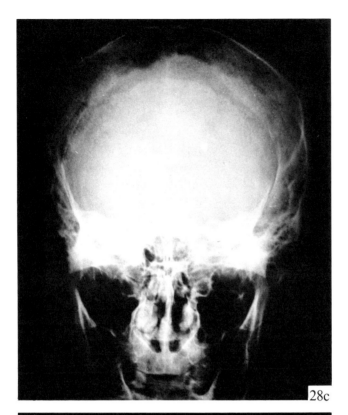

28c

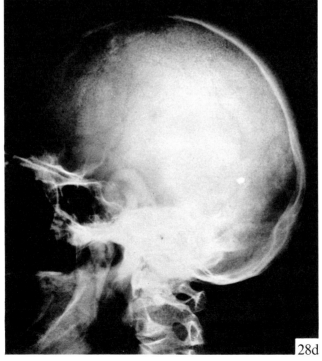

28d

Alternatively, the quadrantic defects extended beyond the horizontal meridian, at least in one monocular field, and involved the quadrant above or below the one primarily affected. Quadrantanopiae with overshooting into the quadrants above or below are represented by cases A-13, A-98, and A-30 (see Figs. 26–28). In two of these cases, A-13 and A-98, the overshooting of the defect is observed for only one eye (see Figs. 26 and 27). All these defects, the partial quadrantanopiae as well as those with overshooting, are characterized by a marked lack of congruence between right and left monocular fields (see below).

A special point of interest regarding quasiquadrantic field defects is their frequent departure from a strictly quadrantic shape, and, more specifically, the tendency towards selective sparing or selective involvement of the horizontal meridian. In a thorough study of visual field defects after penetrating wounds of the visual pathway, Spalding (1952a,b) has recorded several instances of incomplete quadrantanopia in which the defect reached the vertical meridian but fell short of the horizontal. He believes that such defects occur particularly often after wounds implicating the radiation in its anterior portion. Occasionally, however, the effects of lesions in this situation will be the converse: a sector-shaped defect, extending from the periphery towards the fovea and tapering towards the latter, may lie half above and half below the horizontal meridian and consequently obliterate vision along its course (Spalding, 1952a,b).

In the case of occipital lesions (especially those of the occipital poles), Spalding records a relative absence of quadrantic field defects implicating the horizontal meridian. This frequent escape of the horizontal meridian after occipital lesions can be understood by reference to the earlier concept of Henschen (1911), who proposed that the horizontal meridian was represented in a relatively protected situation at the depth of the calcarine fissure, a localization also adopted by Holmes (1918a, 1931, 1934, 1945) and others (e.g., Balado, Adrogue, and Franke, 1928; Spalding, 1952b; Polyak, 1957).

To account for the partial quadrantic defects found after lesions of the anterior radiation, Spalding proposes a revised schema for the disposition of macular and peripheral fibers in that part of the radiation. He believes that it is only in the posterior course of the radiation that macular fibers are completely interposed between the peripheral representations; for the anterior course of the radiation he makes a different assumption. There "the fibers subserving central vision are spread out over the lateral aspect of the radiation, tending to congregate towards the intermediate part, whereas the fibers subserving peripheral vision are spread out on the medial aspect, tending to congregate at the upper and lower margins" (Spalding, 1952a).

This arrangement in the anterior radiation would explain how relatively narrow sector-shaped defects might result from penetrating wounds implicating this part of the radiation; it would also account for the relative frequency of defects reaching the vertical meridian but falling short of the horizontal. Simi-

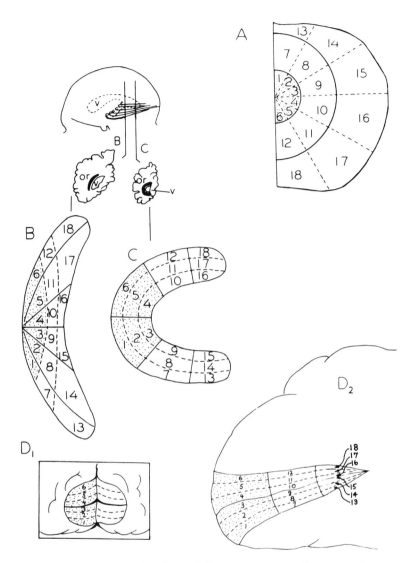

Figure 29. Diagrams suggesting how different sectors and concentric zones of the right homonymous half-field (A) might be represented in the anterior part of the left optic radiation (B), the posterior part of that radiation (C), the lip of the left calcarine fissure (D₁), and the depth of the fissure (D₂). The macular and perimacular regions are indicated by stippling. The two planes of section of the optic radiation (or) in relation to the ventricle (v) are shown schematically in the diagrams on the upper left. Note that the macular fibers in the anterior part of the radiation (plane B) do not completely separate the more peripheral fibers (as postulated by Polyak, 1957), but are here presumed to be concentrated at the lateral margin of the radiation. Only in its posterior part (plane C) does the radiation assume a distribution which conforms to Polyak's view. The numbering of sectors and zones permits one to deduce certain field defects that are not easily reconciled with earlier notions.

Adapted by permission from J. M. K. Spalding, *J. Neurol. Neurosurg. Psychiat.* 15:99–109, 169–183 (1952).

larly, the arrangement would account for the occasional appearance of narrow sector-shaped defects implicating the horizontal meridian in a selective fashion.

By using the numbers in our diagram (Fig. 29), we can illustrate Spalding's hypothesis in some detail. Destruction of the upper third of the anterior radiation (plane B in Fig. 29) could result in a partial lower quadrant defect (primarily of sectors 12, 18, 17) with sparing of the horizontal meridian (see Spalding, 1952a, p. 104). Sector-shaped defects, selectively involving the horizontal meridian, could result from lesions of the anterior radiation in parts of sectors 3, 4, 9, 10, 15, 16.

The arrangement illustrated in Figure 29 is admittedly conjectural and opposed to the traditional view that macular fibers should be interposed, as a discrete bundle, between the peripheral representations throughout the entire antero-posterior course of the optic radiation. The traditional view has been stated most forcefully by Polyak, who adduced histologic evidence derived from his experiments on monkeys with small lesions of the striate cortex and subsequent retrograde degeneration in different parts of the radiation (1932, 1933). More recently (1957), Polyak has added a thorough analysis of the posterior radiation based on clinico-pathologic material.

It is possible, however, as Spalding points out (1952a,b) that the anterior (and intermediate) parts of the radiation present an arrangement different from its posterior portion (see diagram, Fig. 29).

A recent anatomic study (Harman and Teuber, 1959) has, in fact, lent unexpected support to the postulated need for revision of traditional views on man's optic radiation. In their case (Figs. 30a-g), two successive vascular accidents, 17 months apart, destroyed most of the left, and all of the right striate cortex (compare Figs. 30a,b). Only the lips of the left striate cortex, on the side of the earlier, and less massive vascular lesion, were partly spared (compare Figs. 30a,g). The corresponding spared portion of the left lateral geniculate body (Fig. 30c) gave rise to a discrete bundle of presumably "macular" fibers. However, upon leaving the geniculate (Fig. 30d), these fibers distributed themselves rather widely over the entire dorso-ventral extent of the optic radiation (Fig. 30e). Throughout the anterior and intermediate course of the radiation, these fibers remained dispersed, but they recongregated, as might be expected, just before entering the striate cortex (Figs. 30f,g). This anatomic distribution is not incompatible with the view that fibers representing the upper and lower peripheral quadrants may be concentrated respectively at the lower and upper margins of the optic radiation. However, the macular fibers seem to overlap these peripheral representations over a rather wide extent of the radiation, especially in its anterior and intermediate course.

These observations thus lend rather direct support to the claim that our views on the optic radiation in man may require revision, a revision suggested indirectly by the shapes of the field defects after gunshot wound, as recorded by Spalding (1952a) and by ourselves. If the radiation is indeed laminated over part of its course, as indicated in the diagram (Fig. 29), one could account for the occasional appearance of sector-shaped scotomata following penetrating wounds of the optic radiation. The diagram finds further support from the effects of anterior temporal lobectomies undertaken in the hope of relieving epilepsy (Falconer and Wilson, 1958; Van Buren and Baldwin, 1958). Following such unilateral resections, visual field defects tend to appear, as expected, in the contralateral upper quadrants; with the slightest defect, the loss appears immediately adjacent to the vertical meridian; with larger defects the loss spreads in sector-shaped fashion towards, and with still larger defects beyond, the horizontal meridian (Falconer and Wilson, 1958). Nevertheless, certain difficulties remain.[2]

According to Spalding's proposal, sector-shaped scotomata should either tend to spare the homonymous horizontal meridians, or they should tend to involve these meridians selectively. We did observe scotomata of both kinds, but in most of these cases, the selective sparing or selective involvement of the horizontal meridian was found in one eye and not in the other (e.g., case A-182, Fig. 24). This observation is only a special instance of the frequent lack of congruence between homonymous fields, a problem which we shall discuss in the next section. As we shall see, none of the currently available hypotheses about the anatomy of the visual pathways seem to be adequate, since none can account for the striking lack of congruence we have observed.

---

[2] The results of the two recent studies of anterior temporal resections are discordant in several respects. Falconer and Wilson (1958) report congruent field defects; Van Buren and Baldwin (1958) find defects that were more often incongruent than not. Cushing (1922) had already stressed the lack of congruity of field defects following temporal lobe tumors, and Harrington (1939) attributed these characteristics to a "dissociation in the temporal lobes of homologous fibers from ipsilateral points and their gradual coalescence in the postparietal region." In fact, most of these authors, as well as Duke-Elder (1949), assume that this incongruity decreases the farther back the lesion is situated in the visual pathway, with absolute congruity after lesions in the occipital region. Our own observations are different, since we found departures from congruence after any lesion. A further difficulty is the uncertainty regarding Meyer's loop (Meyer, 1907, 1912; see, also, earlier, Probst, 1906; and, later, Cushing, 1922). Falconer and Wilson (1958) interpret their results as compatible with the prevailing view that the ventral portion of the radiation, in the anterior temporal lobe, loops forward to cap the tip of the ventricle. Van Buren and Baldwin (1958) conclude, in contrast, that this forward-looping is much more limited in extent. It is surprising that neither of these studies bears out the expected correlation between extent of anterior temporal resection and extent of resulting field defect—a correlation made earlier by Penfield in his Hunterian lecture (1954). A great deal will depend, therefore, on anatomic studies of such cases, particularly since the operation itself may not be performed as readily in the future as it has been in the recent past.

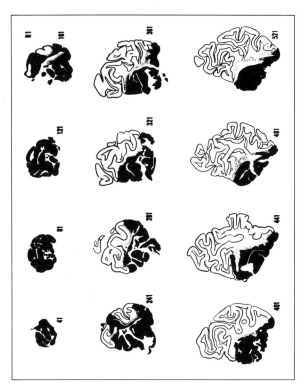

Figures 30a,b. Extent of cerebral destruction (indicated in black) in case M. R. (reported by Harman and Teuber, 1959). Figure 30a (on left) shows effects of a first vascular accident which had been limited to the left hemisphere, producing an incomplete right homonymous hemianopia with partial macular sparing. Note that a portion of the left calcarine cortex (marked cc), near the posterior pole, is preserved. Figure 30b (on right) shows effects of the second vascular accident (17 months after the first, and 7 weeks before death). This second accident involved the right hemisphere and destroyed all of the calcarine cortex on that side. Following this second cerebrovascular accident, the patient complained of total blindness. Optokinetic nystagmus could not be elicited, although pupillary constriction to light was regularly observed. Apparently, this patient did not regain pattern vision during the brief survival period following his second stroke. Nevertheless, blink responses to light could be established by a conditioning procedure (with sound as unconditioned stimulus). These responses were maximal when the stimulus light was directed at the central part of the patient's fields, or slightly to the right; they were not elicited when the light was directed into the left half of his visual field. He continued to complain of his loss of vision until the final week of his life; at that time, he began to deny his blindness and to confabulate visual responses. Such outright denials or confabulations were never observed in our series of field defects due to gunshot wounds (see text, pp. 88–90).

50

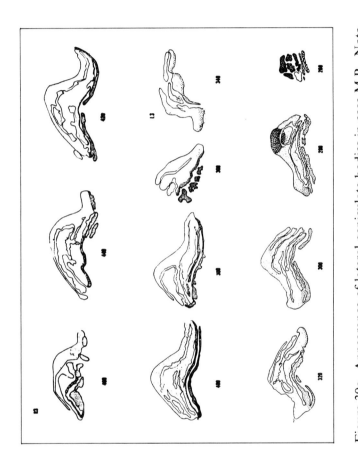

Figure 30c. Appearance of lateral geniculate bodies in case M.R. Note that the right LGB (sections R_3 460, 440, 420, 400, 380, 360) is totally degenerated (the lowermost lamina shows pigmentation). The left LGB (sections L_3 340, 320, 300, 280, 260) shows degeneration except in its dorso-caudal portions (top of sections 280, 260), where there is a spared portion (heavy stippling) corresponding to the part usually considered as representing macular regions in the LGB.

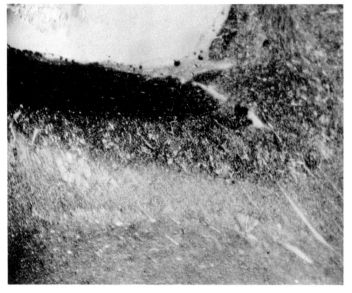

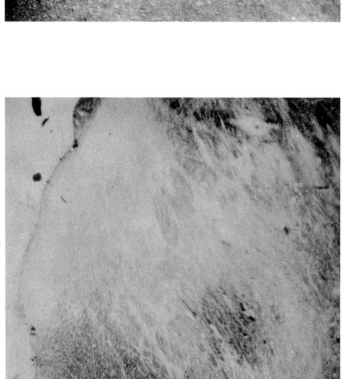

Figure 30d. Left optic radiation of case M.R. in fiber stain (Weigert), just caudal to the left LGB. A bundle of spared fibers can be seen below, and to the left of the center of the microphotograph. This bundle, which corresponds to the spared portion of the LGB, is surrounded by degenerated fibers.

Figure 30e. Left optic radiation, intermediate portions, of case M.R. in fiber stain (Weigert). The spared fibers have spread over the entire dorsoventral extent of the optic radiation. There is a suggestion of a laminated arrangement, with preserved fibers forming a lateral band.

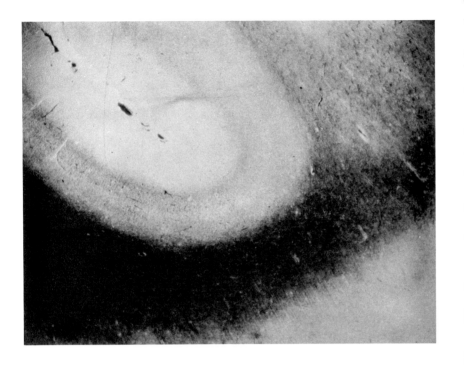

Figure 30g. Preserved portion of calcarine cortex, left cerebral hemisphere, of case M.R. (in Weigert stain). Compare Figure 30a.

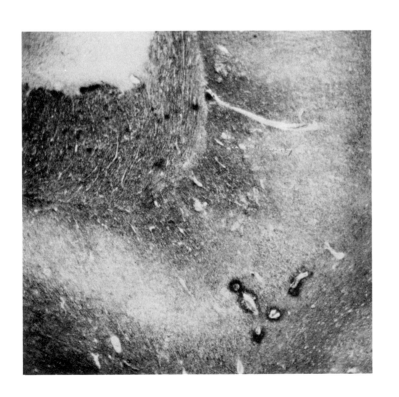

Figure 30f. Left optic radiation of case M.R. in fiber stain (Weigert), just before entering the spared (posterior) portion of the calcarine cortex. Note that the spared fibers recongregate, forming closely adjacent bundles.

6. Shape of Field Defects:
Unexpected Features

According to the classic view of retinocortical projection, corresponding points from homonymous half-retinae are represented in separate laminae of the lateral geniculate body. The fibers representing crossed and uncrossed projections show increasingly precise alignment within the optic radiation. At the level of the striate cortex, the crossed and uncrossed fibers from corresponding retinal points are somehow brought together, either by juxtaposition or discharge into some common element, or both. The functional result of this anatomic convergence is thought to be binocular fusion of corresponding retinal points (e.g., Polyak, 1957). By the same token, lesions in the retrochiasmal visual system should produce field defects which are essentially alike in the monocular fields of the right and the left eye. Some departures from perfect congruence are conceded to result from lesions of the anterior radiation (Wilbrand, 1925–26; Polyak, 1957), but in lesions of the striate cortex the classic view expects "mathematically congruent" field defects (Henschen, 1923; Wilbrand, 1930; Polyak, 1957).

There is one obvious exception to this statement, an exception which is universally admitted (Poppelreuter, 1917; Lenz, 1924): occasionally, retrochiasmal lesions may produce dissimilar field defects in the two eyes by selective destruction, or selective sparing, of that part of the visual pathway which represents the unpaired (purely monocular) portion of the visual field—the so-called monocular crescent. The existence of such defects, which are in effect monocular and hence nonhomonymous, of course does not detract from the claim of congruence for homonymous defects, in other parts of the field. However, there are, in these other parts, true deviations from congruence, and we shall have to ask whether such incongruent defects are not the rule rather than the exception among our cases.

In our experience, homonymous field defects plotted for each eye are similar, but never strictly identical. These departures from congruence are manifested in two ways: (*a*) by an asymmetry in the behavior of homonymous halves of the field depending on whether a field defect is nasal or temporal; (*b*) by a general irregularity in the outline of homonymous scotomata which precludes strict congruence.

Preponderance of Defects in the Nasal Half
of the Visual Field

By definition, homonymous field defects appear, say, on the right side of the right eye and the right side of the left eye. By the same token, the defect in the right eye is in the temporal half of the field, and the one in the left eye, in the nasal half. The same is true, correspondingly, of field defects in the homonymous left half of the field.

Under such conditions the temporal defect will be more obvious to the patient than the homonymous nasal defect, although on plotting the defect in the temporal field usually appears to be smaller and less dense than the one in the nasal field. This temporo-nasal asymmetry accounts for some of the departures from congruence found in homonymous field defects (e.g., cases A-13, A-26, A-29, A-30, A-59, A-66, A-98, A-174, A-182; Figs. 8, 12, 13, 18, 24, 26–28, 31). The extreme instance of such lack of congruence is case A-61 (Figs. 32a,b).

These asymmetries of defects seem to parallel the asymmetry in the fiber spectrum of the optic nerve; as Chacko (1948) has demonstrated, fibers from the nasal retina differ in type (diameter) to some extent from those deriving from the temporal retina. It is also well established that more than half of the fibers from each optic nerve decussate in the human chiasm; possibly only 40 per cent remain uncrossed.

Such anatomic data may be related to the functional predominance of the crossed fibers (representing the temporal half of the field of vision) over the uncrossed fibers (representing the nasal half). Köllner (1914) has shown for the normal adult that the nasal half of each monocular field is relatively neglected. This would account for the patient's greater sensitivity to encroachment upon the temporal half-field. At the same time, the greater cell supply of the temporal representation would make the *perimetric* defect appear smaller on the temporal than on the corresponding nasal side.

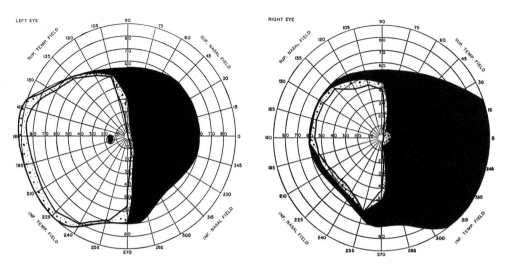

Figure 31a. Case A-59. Right homonymous hemianopia with marked irregularities of the vertical dividing line between spared and affected half-fields. Note the amblyopic margins of the defects, and the partial sparing of the macular region in the right, but not in the left eye. The field defects were caused by a shell-fragment wound of the left occipital region. X-rays reveal a 4 x 4 cm. defect of the left occipital and parietal bones, 4 cm. above the plane of the occipital protuberance. Small bone fragments extended from this wound of entrance in a straight line towards and into the left posterior horn of the ventricle. Fusion thresholds for flickering light were moderately reduced at the fixation point, and more markedly in the periphery of the spared half of the field. Snellen acuity: OS 20/25, OD 20/25.

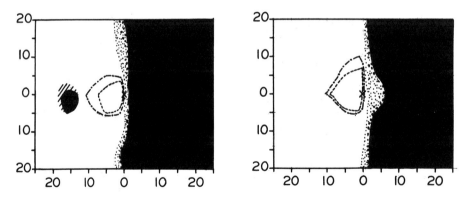

Figure 31b. Central fields obtained for case A-59, showing irregular incongruent outline of the hemianopic defects, and moderate contraction of fields for color. Note, again, the partial sparing of the right lateral half of the macular region in the right eye, but note, also, that this seemingly spared region is amblyopic (indicated by stippling) and that the fields for color fail to show the sparing obtained with the 1° white target.

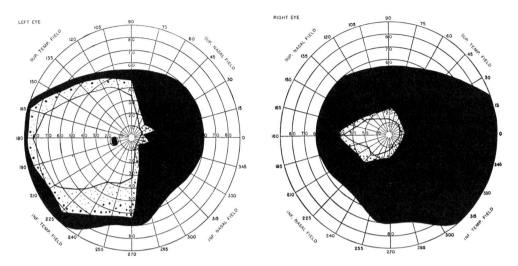

Figure 32a. Case A-61. Extreme instance of incongruence in a case of right homonymous hemianopia with irregular vertical dividing line and marked unilateral contraction of the nasal field in the right eye. These field defects were caused by a shell-fragment wound of the left occipital region. Following debridement, the skull defect measured 10.3 x 7.8 cm. The lower margin of this defect involved the occipital protuberance, and extended horizontally to the left of it; the uppermost margin involved the most posterior part of the left parietal bone. Fusion thresholds for flickering light showed depression at the fovea and a more noticeable depression in all the spared parts of the peripheral fields. Snellen acuity: OS 20/25, OD 20/30.

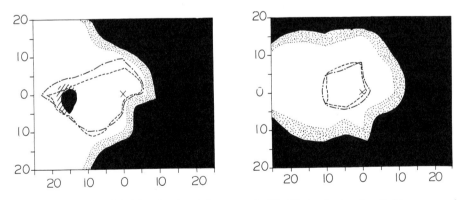

Figure 32b. Central fields obtained for case A-61. Note that color fields are markedly more contracted in the right eye than in the left. Note further that this contraction is asymmetric, being most marked in the right half of the field for OD, and in the right lower quadrants for OD and OS.

The seeming paradox that the same defect appears small in perimetry, and large in the patient's verbal report, is only a special instance of the general dissimilarity between the perimetric field on the one hand, and the functional, or subjective, field on the other (cf. Bender and Teuber, 1946, 1947b, 1948). The wedge-shaped scotomata in macular quadrants, as mentioned earlier, also appear small on perimetry but loom much larger in the patient's everyday visual experience than any peripheral defect which might appear more extensive on perimetry.

Irregularities in Outline of Homonymous Scotomata

Some irregularities in the distribution of fibers from each monocular half-field to the calcarine cortex in the opposite hemisphere will have to be assumed to account for the consistent discrepancies in the outlines of homonymous scotomata (see cases A-71, Fig. 5; A-76, Fig. 10; A-89; A-98, Fig. 27; A-104, Fig. 33; A-109). The defect in each eye is similar to that in the other, but on superimposing the two, certain differences in contour remain. These discrepancies cannot be attributed to shortcomings in the perimetric method, since they remained essentially the same on repeated examination and on fields plotted by different examiners for the same patient. A special instance of such departure from congruence is provided by the differences in the mid-vertical dividing line between the intact and involved sides of the field in cases of hemianopia—the extreme instance being provided again by case A-59 (Fig. 31) where the macula appeared to be spared in one eye, and split in the other.

Such instances of a genuine lack of congruence between homonymous field defects have often been denied (cf. Polyak, 1957), at least for lesions in the occipital lobe. It is just for this reason that we insist on the rather frequent occurrence of such incongruent field defects. We must reject the assumption that these instances of incongruence reflect inaccurate plotting (Wilbrand, 1930; Polyak, 1957).

Inaccurate plotting, where it does occur, tends to be schematic: the less-experienced or less critical examiner introduces straight outlines and sharp transitions from seeing to blind areas in situations where neither might be correct. Furthermore, he often charts the second monocular field while referring to the first. In this fashion, he records perfect congruence, because he anticipates that such congruence should exist, and not because it is really there.

It should be noted that marked departures from congruence can be found in the perimetric fields plotted by Inouye and his colleagues (1909) in their careful studies of Japanese soldiers with cerebral gunshot wounds sustained in the War of 1904–05 (see especially Inouye's cases 12–14, 21; his Figs. 20–22, 34); of particular interest is his case 21, which shows a right homonymous hemianopia with macular sparing in the right eye and a macular scotoma "bulging" into the temporal half of the field in the left eye (*loc. cit.*, p. 81).

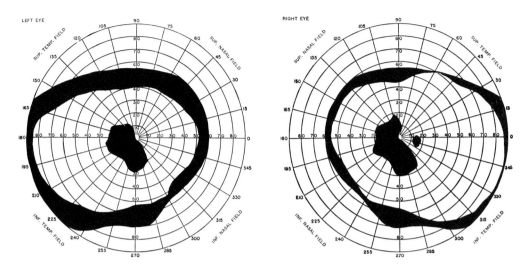

Figure 33. Case A-104. Incongruent insular scotomata primarily involving the left homonymous macular and perimacular regions. These field defects resulted from a shell-fragment wound of the right occipital region. X-rays showed a 2 x 3 cm. oval defect, not covered by plate, in the right occipital bone; the longer axis extended horizontally in the plane of the occipital protuberance, so that the medial margins of the defect touched the midline, with the lateral margins at a distance of 3 cm. to the right. Snellen acuity: OS 20/200, OD 20/50, corrected by glasses to 20/25 OU. In the seventh year after his injury the patient developed transient episodes of distorted vision coincident with swelling and tenderness in the area of the occipital bone defect. These attacks are described in detail in the text, pp. 106–109.

Similarly, one sees numerous incongruent field defects in Poppelreuter's series of 50 cases from the first World War (Poppelreuter, 1917; e.g., pp. 43, 46, 55, 58, fields 16, 19, 30, 32). In these cases, again, the plotting was done with particular care. If we take these results together with our own and those of Marie and Chatelin (1915), we must conclude that the geniculo-calcarine system does not show the reputedly perfect alignment of those elements which mediate corresponding points of the homonymous half-retinae. Somehow, the cortical cell populations belonging to the homonymous halves of the two fields remain at least partly distinct from each other.

Such an arrangement is contrary to that postulated by the checkerboard theory of Wilbrand (1925–26), who believed that crossed and uncrossed elements terminate in the same layer of the cortex, intermingled in a precise alternating pattern like the black and white squares of a checkerboard. Perfect mathematical congruence was thought to result from this scheme. Since the scotomata do not show this postulated congruence, crossed and uncrossed representations may be partly displaced from each other within the same cortical layers, or may be found at different depths of the striate cortex. The most plastic expression of the latter view is the attribution of uncrossed projections to lamina IVa and of the more numerous crossed projections to lamina IVc of the striate cortex; the intervening layer, IVb, corresponding to the stripe of Gennari, is thought to provide in some manner the required binocular fusion (Kleist, 1926; the arrangement was considered by Bárány, 1924, but rejected in favor of a postulated ending of crossed and uncrossed elements at different depths of IVc, with the stria of Gennari again acting as a mixing zone).

All of these assumptions, so far, remain hypothetical, since there is neither histologic nor physiologic proof of the postulated independent termination of crossed and uncrossed fibers at different depths of the striate cortex (see Sholl, 1955, 1956). Such an arrangement, however, would be consistent with the lack of congruence of homonymous scotomata, a point already taken by Kleist (1926) and reiterated by Balado, Malbran, and Franke (1934), who attempted to prove by autopsy that the laminar arrangement suggested by Kleist does in fact account for lack of congruence of field defects after sub-total destruction of the striate cortex. We believe that ultimate proof can be obtained only by modern physiologic methods, such as micro-electrode recording at different depths of the cortex (Jung, 1958; Hubel, 1959) or selective laminar destruction by heavy ionizing particles (Malis, Loevinger, Kruger, and Rose, 1957).

Nonhomonymous Defects

Despite the preponderance of homonymous (though incongruent) field defects after retrochiasmal lesions, the occasional appearance of nonhomonymous defects in these cases should not be overlooked. Such nonhomonymous defects arise most readily in the area of the monocular crescent, i.e., that portion of the peripheral field on the temporal side of each eye which extends from about 60° to about 90° (Fig. 34). In this portion of the field, vision is mediated through only one eye: for the left peripheral crescent through the left eye, and for the right crescent, through the right eye. The corresponding portion of the retina lies on the nasal side, owing to inversion of the visual field by the lens of the eye, and the fibers originating from that portion all cross into the opposite hemisphere. As a result, a lesion of the hemisphere which destroys the representation of the crescent is manifested by a monocular defect, which is thus not only incongruent but nonhomonymous.

Selective involvement or selective sparing of a monocular crescent was observed during World War I in cases of missile wounds (see Fleischer, 1916, case 1; Poppelreuter, 1917; Riddoch, 1917; Holmes, 1919a). In these instances the temporal half-moon (from 60° to 90°) was lost, as in case H (group SD, Fig. 35), or preserved, as in case C (group SD, Fig. 21). Such defects were considered compatible with the assumption that the extreme periphery of the field projects most anteriorly into the depth of the calcarine fissure; nevertheless, from what has been said before, it remains difficult to understand how an injury there could remain restricted to one side, or how it

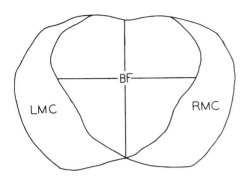

Figure 34. Diagram of the normal extent of the visual fields, showing the monocular crescents, that is, those lateral portions from 60° to 90° in the periphery of the temporal fields which are seen only through corresponding eyes. These monocular crescents are represented by fibers which are entirely crossed, so that they are represented unilaterally, each in its cerebral hemisphere. LMC = left monocular crescent; RMC = right monocular crescent; BF = binocular field.

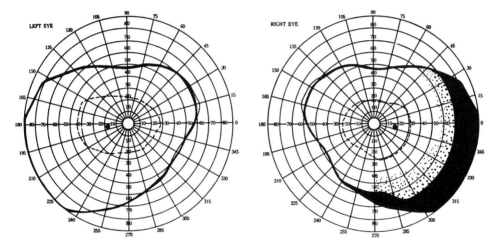

Figure 35. Case SD-H. Selective involvement of a monocular crescent (in this case, in the right eye), probably the residual of an initial right homonymous hemianopia. This defect was recorded approximately four months following a shell-fragment wound in the left occipito-parietal area. The injury was complicated by another and smaller lesion in the right parietal lobe, where the patient had been struck a few minutes before he sustained the major injury to the left posterior lobe substance. This patient exhibited marked "extinction" on double simultaneous stimulation in the visual fields. While fixating on a central point, he clearly perceived the form and color of an object placed in his right field of vision. However, when another object was brought into view on his left side, the image on the right became invisible to him, or became blurred and dull. As soon as the stimulus on the left was removed, the object on the right side appeared to be normal. For further details on these phenomena, see text, pp. 78, 83–84 and Figure 45.

could spare radiation fibers as they pass around the posterior horn of the ventricle.

At times crescentic defects have therefore been ascribed to lesions of radiation rather than cortex, in keeping with the proposed segregation of fibers in the radiation (see above) which allot uppermost and lowermost portions to the representation of the extreme periphery. From this scheme, the defect to be expected should be quadrantic—the upper half of a crescent after destruction of the lower border of the radiation, and the lower half of a crescent after destruction of the upper border.[3] Selective loss or sparing of half-crescents has indeed been observed (see especially Poppelreuter, 1917), but the difficulties of understanding the whole crescents remain. Simultaneous damage to upper and lower borders of the radiation are conceivable, but in the absence of histologic proof such lesions seem rather unlikely.

Before leaving the problem of grossly dissimilar defects in right and left fields, we should point out that one occasionally encounters nonhomonymous scotomata due to simultaneous damage to retina and brain (see Marie and Chatelin, 1916a). One of our cases (A–102, Fig. 6) illustrates such a combination of lesions. In this case a rupture of the chorioid in one eye, possibly sustained simultaneously with the trauma of the posterior lobe of the brain, added a conspicuous scotoma, limited to one eye, to the other field defects traceable to the occipital lesions.

THE PROBLEM OF MACULAR SPARING

The departures from congruence of homonymous defects modify but do not deny the principle of orderly retinotopical projection. Nor does selective involvement (or sparing) of monocular crescents detract from the principle as long as one assumes that structures representing the crescent can be selectively destroyed or preserved. A much more serious issue is raised by the frequent escape of macular vision following extensive injury to one occipital lobe or optic radiation. The phenomenon of macular sparing has been noted particularly in cases of hemianopia after vascular accidents, and the controversy about the anatomic or functional interpretation of such macular sparing is as old as the use of perimetry for the plotting of visual fields (Förster, 1867).

---

[3] By referring to the diagrams in Figure 29, it can be seen how lesions of the posterior radiation (plane C) could readily result in selective destruction or sparing of lower or upper half of a peripheral crescent (e.g., destruction or sparing of sectors 16, 17, 18 in plane C). At the level of the striate cortex (D_1, D_2), the diagrams suggest why partial destruction frequently produces zonal field defects, or defects with extensions in the form of bays, partial rings, or claws: a band of destruction reaching through sectors 7–12 in D_2 would result in a scotoma shaped like a half-ring in A; a defect involving sections 13–18 in D_2 would analogously produce a crescent scotoma in A. However, all of the difficulties mentioned in the text (p. 60) remain. It must also be stressed that the diagrams of Figure 29 are based on conjecture. They are included for the sake of exposition, and in order to guide neuropathologic studies which alone can settle these issues.

This sparing of the macula has led at times to the belief that the principle of retinotopical projection may not apply to the macular part of the field. The macular fibers and cell bodies were assumed to be diffused throughout the striate cortex (Brouwer, 1917; Foerster, 1929); doubly represented, i.e., each homonymous half of the macula projected into *both* occipital lobes (Wilbrand, 1881, 1895; Heine, 1900; Pfeifer, 1925, 1930); or mediated by a striate and some supplementary, extra-striate focus (Hyndman, 1939). We shall see that, while macular sparing remains a problem (see Fox and German, 1936; Halstead, Walker, and Bucy, 1940), its solution may require less radical assumptions than might at first appear.

A careful inspection of the visual fields in our series, with special regard for macular sparing or its absence, reveals, first, that sparing occurs in many instances, and second, that it happens under such a variety of conditions that any single interpretation appears inadequate. In particular, our observations detract from the view that macular sparing should invariably occur with lesions in one situation (e.g., in the occipital lobe), and never with lesions in another (e.g., the optic tract).

Hemianopia resulting from a gunshot wound of one occipital region may lead occasionally to macular splitting, that is, the dividing line between blind and seeing halves of the field passes through the fixation point. Such splitting of the macula is illustrated by case A-82 (Fig. 22b). The particularly detailed surgical notes suggest that the lesion was in the right occipital lobe; there are no indications that the optic tract (rather than the geniculostriate system) might have been implicated. The macula appeared split on the campimeter for color, form, and motion of the target. This case raises additional doubts about the alleged observation that macular sparing should occur regularly with lesions of the occipital lobe.

There is likewise little question that small wedge-shaped scotomata in the macular region may reach the fixation point (e.g., cases A-66, Fig. 8, and A-76, Fig. 10; see also Marie and Chatelin, 1915; Moreau, 1918, especially case II; Symonds, 1945; and Spalding, 1952b); in several of these instances the entrance wound of the missile was definitely at the occipital protuberance (e.g., our case A-76, Fig. 10).

A second instance of macula-splitting hemianopia was manifested by a casualty of the Korean campaign (case AK-8). The nature of the lesion was such that involvement of the posterior radiation seemed not unlikely. However, in a third instance of macular splitting, a shell fragment had passed through the occipital protuberance, resulting in a pinpoint scotoma (1° across) at 2° from the fixation point in the homonymous right half-fields (case A-48, Figs. 36a,b). At the same time this patient exhibited a macula-splitting right hemiamblyopia, manifested primarily as a deficit for color discrimination (hemiachromatopsia).

These three cases are in contrast with the 15 other cases of hemianopia or hemiamblyopia in group A; all 15 showed varying degrees of sparing of

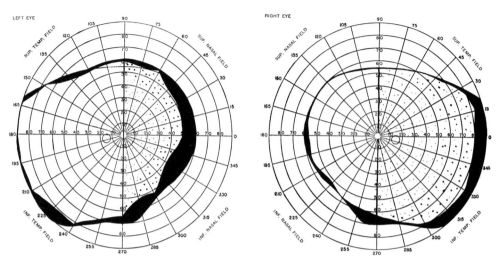

Figure 36a. Case A-48. Right homonymous hemiamblyopia, apparently macula-splitting and most prominently manifested in the form of a right homonymous defect in color discrimination, due to penetration of the left occipital region by flak. The injury produced a 2.7 x 3 cm. defect in the left occipital bone; the lower margin of the defect was found to lie 5 cm. above the occipital protuberance, the upper margin was in the posterior part of the left parietal bone. A small metallic foreign body was removed from the brain substance in this region on the day of the wounding, but x-rays later disclosed a bone fragment 3 x 8 mm. in the left parieto-occipital lobe, 2 cm. anterior and inferior to the center of the bone defect. Traditionally, such a defect would be designated as a hemiachromatopia. However, the impairment was not specific for the discrimination of colors, since acuity in the right homonymous halves of the fields was also diminished, fusion thresholds for flickering light were markedly reduced, and dark adaptation was correspondingly impaired in that region. There also were marked fluctuation and obscuration in the affected part of the visual field. For this reason the hemiamblyopia was more disturbing to this patient than an outright hemianopia.

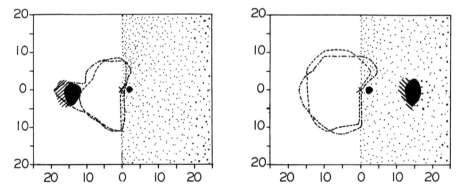

Figure 36b. Central fields obtained for case A-48, showing right homonymous hemiamblyopia and hemiachromatopia. In each field, a pinpoint scotoma, less than 2° in diameter, lies just to the right of the fixation point.

macular vision on the involved side of the field. A characteristic instance is furnished by case A-86 (Figs. 37a,b)—a patient with right homonymous hemianopia who nevertheless could perceive color, form, and motion of 1° and ½° targets as far as 2.5° to the right of his fixation point.

The perimetric and campimetric fields, however, reveal an additional feature in this case: the normal blind spot was consistently shifted laterally towards the blind side, and this displacement amounted to 3°—more than is needed to explain the apparent sparing of central vision. The same displacement of the blind spot can be noted in case A-28 (Figs. 38a,b), A-70, and A-100 (Figs. 40a,b); in all these, part of the macula seemed to be spared, not only for form, but also for color, i.e., the color fields extended into the implicated halves of the fields. In these cases, the sparing of the (anatomic) hemifovea is thus apparent rather than real. We are dealing with the interesting phenomenon of persistent extra-foveal fixation: the appearance of a pseudo-fovea (see Fuchs, 1922; and below).

In some of the remaining cases (A-59, Figs. 31a,b; A-61, Figs. 32a,b), the dividing line between blind and seeing portions of the field is highly irregular; here the blind spot is not shifted from its normal position, and the macula seems truly spared. Yet, the sparing is not complete: while the macular field seems intact for form and motion of targets, it is split for color (see case A-59, Fig. 31b, campimetric field). Hence, the hemifovea *is* impaired in these cases, though to a lesser degree than other, more peripheral portions of the implicated portion of the field.

Again, sparing is not an all-or-none affair, but seems related to irregularities in the outline of the defect. This is further underscored by the particularly puzzling case, A-59, in which the macula seemed to be spared (but *not* for color) in one eye, and split in the other eye (Figs. 31a,b).

The most parsimonious interpretation of all these findings would appear to be as follows: apparent macular sparing is due to a combination of four factors (*a*) slight irregularities of fixation during perimetry (see Keen and Thomson, 1871); (*b*) persistent pseudo-foveae (see below); (*c*) lack of congruence between the monocular fields (see above); or (*d*) lower vulnerability of central as against peripheral fields, owing to the widespread macular representation in optic radiation and cortex and, possibly, to better vascular supply of the cortical macula.

The last factor—the better vascular supply of the cortical representation of the macular region—was suggested by the inventor of the perimeter, Richard Förster. In 1867, Förster stressed the frequent occurrence of macular sparing in cases of hemianopia. In 1890, he proposed that "in case the principal vessel of the occipital lobe is obstructed and an extensive area of the cortex is shut off, precisely that portion of the cortex which corresponds to the most acute vision may be spared" (R. Förster, 1890, p. 106; see also autopsy of Förster's case by Sachs, 1895). A similar solution for the problem

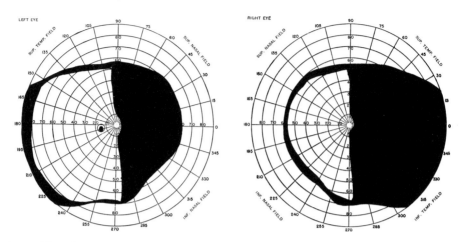

Figure 37a. Case A-86. Right homonymous hemianopia with rather marked sparing of the central region; this sparing, however, seems to be due to a consistent shift in fixation, apparent from the central field charts (Fig. 37b), which show displacement of the normal blind spot downward and 2–3° to the right. The injury which caused these field defects was produced by shell fragments which entered the left posterior parietal area. The skull defect is now covered by a 6 x 4 cm. tantalum plate. On the day of wounding bone fragments and metallic foreign bodies were recovered from a track extending from the cranial defect into the brain; the track measured approximately 2 cm. in diameter and at least 12 cm. in length, and crossed the midline on an oblique course. The posterior part of the parietal lobe was thus damaged on both the left and the right side. Snellen acuity: OS 20/40, OD 20/40.

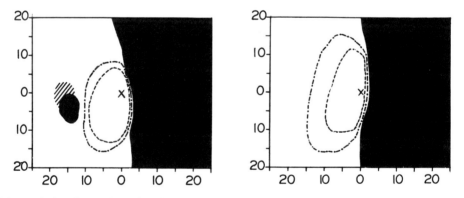

Figure 37b. Central fields obtained for case A-86, showing right homonymous hemianopia and apparent macular sparing. The normal blind spot is displaced 4–5° downward and 2–3° laterally to the right. This shift apparently accounts for the 2° sparing of vision to the right of the fixation point and is consistent with the presence of a new, or pseudo-fovea. Note the moderate contraction of color fields.

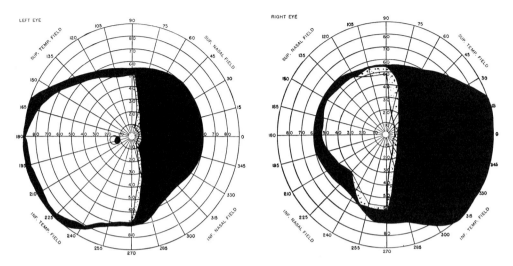

Figure 38a. Case A-28. Right homonymous hemianopia with irregular dividing line displaced somewhat to the right from the midvertical meridian. Note the corresponding displacement of the normal blind spot to the right. This defect resulted from penetration, by shell fragments, of the left fronto-temporo-parietal regions. On the day after the injury, metal and bone fragments were removed from a huge gaping wound, and a branch of the middle cerebral artery was ligated.

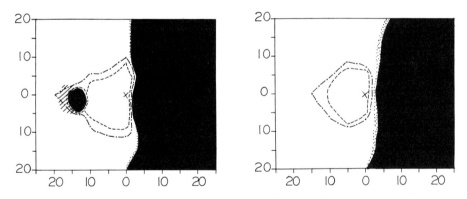

Figure 38b. Central fields obtained for case A-28, showing irregular outline of the right homonymous hemianopia, as well as lateral displacement of the normal blind spot to the right by 2–3°. This may account for the sparing of parts of the central field.

presented by genuine sparing, particularly in cases of double hemianopia (see Rønne, 1914), was suggested by Holmes and Lister in 1916, who considered the pole of the occipital lobe to be at the "watershed" of the posterior and middle cerebral arteries, and hence thought that it may "under conditions draw blood from both, and if one is blocked, the other may suffice to maintain its nutrition" (Fig. 39). Polyak (1957) has presented a great deal of anatomic data to support these views.

We believe that the factors we have listed may account for the various forms of apparent as well as genuine macular sparing, especially after lesions of the occipital lobe. Taken together, these factors make it unnecessary to adopt Wilbrand's famous notion of bilateral central representation for the macula (Wilbrand, 1881, 1895; Heine, 1900). In particular, there is no reason to believe that radiation fibers cross somewhere in their more posterior course through the splenium of the corpus callosum to reach the opposite occipital lobe (Lenz, 1924, 1927; Pfeifer, 1925, 1930; Penfield, Evans, and MacMillan, 1935; for review, see Putnam and Liebman, 1942). This anatomic assumption is paralleled by the long-standing belief that macular sparing occurs with lesions of striate cortex or posterior radiations, and splitting with those of anterior radiations or optic tract.

Actually, macula-splitting hemianopiae were found in one-third of all tumors of the occipital lobe in Allen's review (1930) from the National Hospital in London. Bender and Kanzer (1939) stressed the absence of any correlation between macular splitting or macular sparing on the one hand, and the site of the lesion in the radiation or striate cortex on the other. Finally, Austin, Lewey, and Grant (1949), on the basis of a series of cases, showed that central vision was spared as often after occipital lobectomy as after chiasmal lesions. The anatomic assumption of a crossed callosal bundle, ad hoc from the start, is incompatible with the results of unilateral occipital lobectomy in the monkey (Polyak, 1933) and in man (Putnam, 1926a,b; Polyak, 1957), where degeneration is confined to the lateral geniculate body on the same side. Similarly, degeneration in the contralateral geniculate does not follow transection of one optic radiation. Most telling in this respect is one of Polyak's cases, in which the patient exhibited a macula-splitting right hemianopia. At autopsy destruction of the left optic radiation as well as the splenium of the corpus callosum was traced to a neoplasm but no degeneration was found in the right lateral geniculate. Such findings provide rather definite evidence against the existence of a "crossed callosal bundle" of macular fibers.

There is additional negative evidence. The callosal bundle, postulated by Lenz and described by Pfeifer (1925), was restudied in Brouwer's laboratory by Putnam (1926a,b), who concluded that these fibers actually did not cross into the opposite hemisphere but ended, after a circuitous course, in the homolateral occipital lobe. This finding was confirmed subsequently by Krainer (1936) and Krainer and Suwa (1936). Similarly, section of the callosal splenium does not interfere with the macular sparing which can be found after

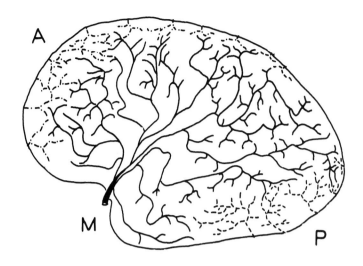

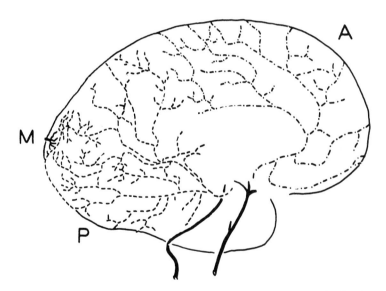

Figure 39. Schematic drawings showing vascular supply to the brain: lateral view (above) and medial view of left hemisphere (below). Distribution of the anterior cerebral artery (A) is indicated by dots and dashes (_._.); of the middle cerebral artery (M) by continuous lines (_____); and of the posterior artery (P) by dashes (____). The diagrams show how the occipital regions just above the pole receive vessels from middle *and* posterior arteries, an arrangement which might account for some forms of sparing of the macular regions of the visual field.

Adapted by permission from S. Polyak, *The Vertebrate Visual System* (University of Chicago Press, 1957).

subtotal amputation of one occipital lobe (Hyndman, 1939). Lack of decussations above the level of the geniculate body was suggested by an ingenious experiment in the monkey (Maison, Settlage, and Grether, 1939) which combined amputation of one occipital lobe with section of the opposite optic tract; the animal appeared to be totally blind following these procedures.

However strong the evidence against supra-geniculate decussation, phenomena of macular sparing continue to present difficulties for the principle of antero-posterior projection. Extensive amputations of one occipital lobe are not infrequently followed by some return of contralateral macular vision; in most of these cases some striate cortex at the depth of the fissure may have remained (especially in the cases of Penfield, Evans, and MacMillan, 1935). If such remnants of (anterior) striate cortex play a role, we would be hard put to maintain the principle of peripheral projection to anterior parts of the calcarine fissure, and macular projection to posterior parts. It is conceivable, however, that such remnants of tissue merely play a role in establishing a pseudo-fovea, which we believe leads to apparent rather than real macular sparing. Even the most rigorous control of eye movements during perimetry, as in the study by Halstead, Walker, and Bucy (1940), does not preclude the sort of pseudo-sparing we have attributed to the formation of a vicarious fovea; control of fixation is best achieved by plotting the normal blind spot in relation to the fixation point.

In spite of all these arguments the return of some macular vision in cases of bilateral hemianopia remains a problem for any anatomic view, as we have pointed out earlier. The problem is underscored by those cases in which the most posterior portions of the calcarine region are presumed to have been removed bilaterally during surgery, as in McGavic's case 6 (McGavic, 1947), a case which is unfortunately described much too briefly. A full study, anatomic as well as clinical, of such a case would seem to us to be more important than continued study of the less paradoxical macular sparing, following unilateral resection of the occipital lobe (Balado and Malbran, 1932; Horrax and Putnam, 1932; Fox and German, 1936; see also the excellent critical review of these problems by Putnam and Liebman, 1942).

One final source of macular sparing remains to be considered. Contrary to Polyak (1957) we do not believe that present-day histologic evidence excludes the possibility of some intermingling of right and left macular fibers in the neuroretina, or further up in the optic chiasm. Some irregularities in the course of these and other fibers is in any event rather likely if one considers the nature of embryonic development in the visual and other neural systems.

In consonance with this assumption of somewhat irregular growth is the observation that the vertical dividing line between blind and intact halves of a hemianopic field is rarely straight. We have only one case (A-8) in which a straight line is approximated; all others show dividing lines which curve in or out, departing more or less markedly from a straight line (cases A-28, Figs. 38a, b; A-61, Figs. 32a,b; A-86, Figs. 37a,b; and especially A-100, Figs. 40a,b).

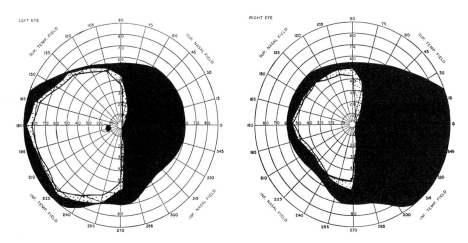

Figure 40a. Case A-100. Right homonymous hemianopia with irregular vertical dividing line and displaced blind spot (to the right). These field defects were caused by a shell-fragment wound in the left occipital region, about 3 cm. above the protuberance, with fracture lines extending laterally and obliquely upwards into the temporal and parietal lobes. Fusion thresholds for flickering light were found to be reduced in the peripheral portion of the spared (left) homonymous half-fields. Snellen acuity: OS 20/25, OD 20/40.

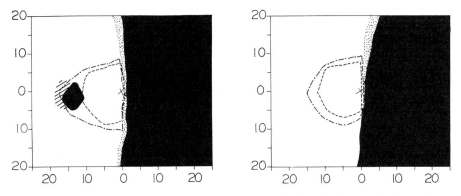

Figure 40b. Central fields obtained for case A-100, showing irregular boundary of the right homonymous hemianopia. The lateral shift of the normal blind spot to the right is indicative of the existence of a pseudo-fovea.

Similar observations were made earlier by Poppelreuter (1917) with his studies of gunshot wound cases of World War I. Poppelreuter attributed these deviations from a straight line to postulated irregularities in the chiasmal course of fibers crossing from either side of the midvertical meridian of the retina.

COLOR FIELDS

In its strongest form (Henschen, 1911), the principle of retinotopical projection implies that homonymous field defects should be (a) congruent in the two eyes, and (b) identical under different conditions of testing. Neither of these two requirements is met in our series of cases. We have shown that homonymous field defects depart from strict congruence: a glance at the visual fields we have presented will indicate that defects can vary in outline as test conditions are changed. In a number of cases, the area of blindness is less extensive for moving than for stationary targets (a phenomenon that will be discussed below). Even more obvious is the difference between fields plotted for white and for colored targets. That this difference should exist is not surprising, if one considers the analogous situation in the normal field of vision. In the extreme periphery of the normal field, stationary white targets rapidly "fade out," but can be reported as soon as they are set in motion. Farther inward, normal subjects can discriminate presence from absence of the stationary white target, but one has to go still farther towards the central field before a subject can reliably distinguish different, colored targets. The extent of these "fields for color" has been determined by Ferree and Rand (1919) and others; they vary in diameter, depending primarily on the nature of the hues employed, the number of different hues to be discriminated, and the angular size of the colored targets. When number of hues and size of targets are held constant, the area in which red can be distinguished from gray is larger in diameter than the area for green (Ferree and Rand, *loc. cit;* Traquair, 1949). The same conditions obtain in defective fields, but they show additional features which force us to qualify the principle of retinotopical projection.

Concave Contours of Fields for Color

The most important feature of fields for colored targets is their tendency to duplicate, at a smaller scale, the outline of the peripheral field. Thus, an incomplete quadrant defect for form and motion, in the extreme periphery, is usually associated with a corresponding contraction of the color fields, closer to the center, in the same quadrant. Occasionally a field may show a quadrantanopia for form, but a hemianopia for color. In such instances (e.g., case A-30, Figs. 28a,b) the early post-traumatic history reveals an initial complete hemianopia. Of particular interest are fields in which a slight indentation in the outline of the color fields is the last remnant of an earlier quadrantic defect for form and motion (see case SD-S, Fig. 41).

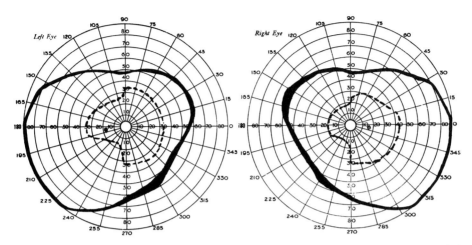

Figure 41. Case SD-S. Homonymous contraction of fields for color (1° red) in the left half-fields. The contraction in the contour of the color field was a residual of an initial left homonymous hemianopia following a shell-fragment wound of the right occipito-parietal region. Note that the contraction is more marked in the left lower quadrants (in which the field defects lasted longer) than in the left upper quadrants. Note also that the contraction is greater in the nasal half of the field (right eye) than in the temporal half (left eye).

Reproduced by permission from M. B. Bender and H.-L. Teuber, *Arch. Neurol. Psychiat.* 58:721–739 (1947).

Eccentric Position of Color Fields

As has been pointed out much earlier (Inouye, 1909; Poppelreuter, 1917), careful plotting of color fields in cases of hemianopia or of macular scotoma may reveal color fields that are eccentric relative to their normal position. A particularly striking instance is furnished by case SD-B (Fig. 7).

Macula-Splitting Color Defects: Hemiachromatopia

Inability to discriminate the colors of small targets can exist in homonymous half-fields as a seemingly isolated disturbance—that is, isolated as long as one does not search for other perceptual deficits. Such a hemiachromatopia is illustrated by our case A-48 (Figs. 36a,b). In this case the defect for color is definitely macula-splitting (see Szily's case 28, 1918, nearly identical to ours!). It must be stressed, however, with regard to case A-48, as well as case SD-S, that our results do not support the older concept (e.g., Wilbrand, 1881; Best, 1920) of selective disturbance in color discrimination per se. As we have pointed out elsewhere, such cases show characteristic patterns of change; their deficit in color discrimination is only one among several symptoms, including reduced fusion thresholds for flickering light (e.g., case A-48, Fig. 42), altera-

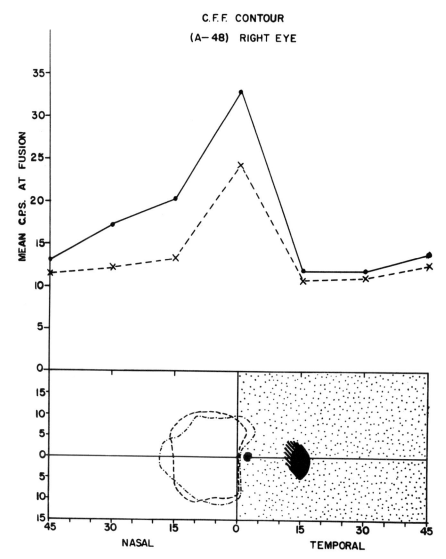

Figure 42. Flicker fusion contours obtained for case A-48 (see Figs. 36a,b). The campimetric field is shown below. The ordinates in the upper part of the figure give the number of flashes per second at which the flickering light appeared fused. Note that thresholds are highest in the fovea. Note that the depression of thresholds in the affected (right) half-field is more marked for the 2° target (_____) than for the 30″ target (– – – –). For details, see text, pp. 92–94 and Figs. 48–49.

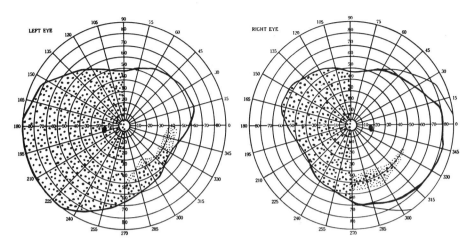

Figure 43a. Case SD-Me. Left homonymous hemiamblyopia with irregular exten-sion into the right lower quadrants. In this case a shell fragment traversed the right midparietal region and entered the third ventricle. The patient presented curious dysesthesiae in the affected half of his field, as described in text.

tion in dark adaptation (Krieger and Bender, 1949), and similar changes (Bender and Teuber, 1949; Teuber and Bender, 1949).

Special Forms of Disordered Color Perception in
Hemiamblyopia: Visual Dysesthesiae

An analogous grouping of symptoms can be demonstrated in those cases of hemiamblyopia, in which color sensations seem to be perverted rather than lost (see Poppelreuter, 1917). In our case SD-Me (Figs. 43a–e), all colors ex-posed to the amblyopic (left) half of the field impressed the patient as being "muddy," or rather "indescribable." It proved, in fact, impossible to obtain matches between identical or different color mixtures (on a color wheel) shown alternately to the affected and unaffected halves of the field. At the same time, all visual stimuli impinging on the impaired half-field tended to elicit exaggerated startle-reactions (see Furlow, Bender, and Teuber, 1947; Bender, Furlow, and Teuber, 1949). The patient insisted that everything visible to him on his left had a disagreeable quality, quite unlike anything in the less impaired, right half of the field.

This curious complaint formed part of a more general hemisensory syn-drome, in which tactile or auditory stimulation on the left led likewise to fre-quent defensive reactions, and was described either as unbearable or, less often, as abnormally "soothing." Such a change in the quality of sensations opposite a deep cerebral lesion has often been reported (under the designation of "thalamic syndrome," Déjérine and Roussy, 1906; Head, 1920), but previous accounts of such cases do not refer to analogous perversion of visual sensations in the hemiamblyopic fields. Despite these unusual features, however, case SD-Me corresponded closely to A-48 in that there was marked reduction in flicker

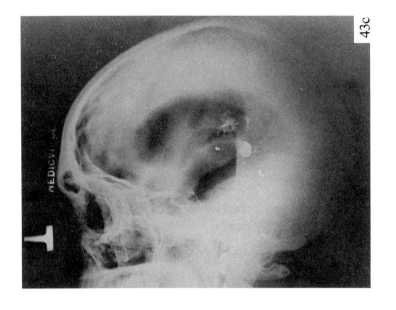

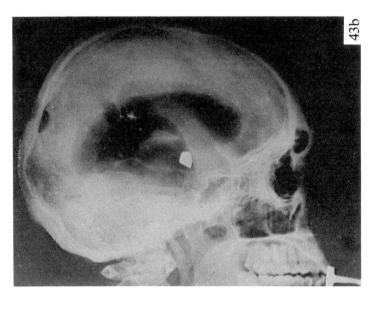

Figures 43b,c. Pneumo-encephalogram (Case SD-Me), showing continual movement of a retained metallic foreign body in a dilated ventricular system with changes in position of the patient's head. In the brow-down position (see on left) the fragment rests at the most anterior end of the third ventricle; in the brow-up position (see on right) the fragment floats to the most posterior portion of the third ventricle.

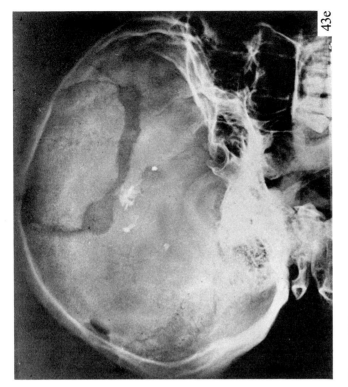

Figure 43d. Same case. Pneumo-encephalogram showing the shell fragment in midline within the third ventricle.

Figure 43e. Same case. X-ray of skull (right lateral view) taken after surgical removal of the intraventricular foreign body. Note the wound of entrance in the right midparietal region and the margins of the large right fronto-parietal osteoplastic flap.

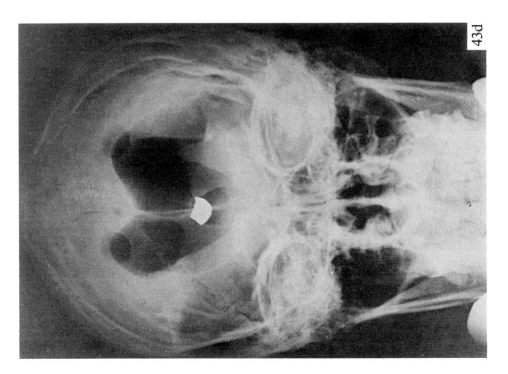

fusion in the affected areas of the field. This persistent deficit indicated that the alteration of color perception in amblyopic regions was only one change among many other, more general changes in visual performance.

Case Me in group SD was unusual in various other respects. The lesion itself (see Figs. 43b–e) was almost unique; a large shell fragment had traversed the right midparietal region and entered the third ventricle, in which it shifted about, with changes in the position of the patient's head. Eleven months after the wounding, a right frontal osteoplastic flap was reflected, and an irregular area of cortex about 45 mm. in diameter was resected down to the lateral ventricle. The foramen of Munro was then slightly enlarged, and the foreign body removed from the third ventricle. Immediately after this procedure, and during the next 8 days, the patient presented a complete hemianopia rather than the hemiamblyopia which had existed before surgery. Then the hemiamblyopia returned, but it now lacked the feature which had been so upsetting to the patient before operation, namely, the visual dysesthesiae. Instead, the patient now showed marked left-sided "extinction," on double simultaneous stimulations of left and right half-fields (see below, pp. 83–84 and Fig. 45). The same change had taken place in the tactile sphere: extinction had supervened, and the left-sided dysesthesiae and paresthesiae had permanently disappeared.

Selectivity of Color Deficits

From the evidence presented, it should be clear that in cases such as SD-Me, or SD-S, or A-48, the apparent regional dissociation of color and form discrimination must not be interpreted as indicating *selective* impairment of color vision as such. True dissociation would require that one function (e.g., color discrimination) be lost in areas where form vision is unchanged. We fully agree with Holmes' view (1918a, 1945) that areas of diminished or absent color discrimination are also areas of diminished acuity (see Henschen, 1910; Marie and Chatelin, 1916b; Monbrun, 1919; Lenz, 1921). Moreover, we have never observed defects which would represent the converse of achromatopia, namely, intact color discrimination combined with serious alteration or loss of form perception. There is thus no evidence for a genuine dissociation (see Teuber, 1955) of color and pattern vision. The different tasks involved in perimetry tap visual performance at different levels of complexity. Seemingly selective impairment of one aspect of vision (e.g., color discrimination) reflects, we believe, a corresponding rank order in the vulnerability of different levels of function, in the presence of lesions in their common substrate.

In terms of retinotopical projection, this means that an area of loss of function is surrounded by areas of diminished or altered function; such graded effects of lesions seem to us incompatible with the strong form of the principle of retinotopical projection, which implies a rigid point-for-point mapping of the visual field into the striate cortex.

Pseudo-Foveae and Other Persistent Changes in Fixation

The observations so far considered may suggest a need for qualifying the principle of retinotopical projection, but nothing as yet has induced us to reject the principle as such. We now have to discuss a group of phenomena which have been considered at times as an outright negation of the principle of consistent projection. These are the instances in which a patient with field defect seemingly "reorganizes" the remaining field around a new fixation point which corresponds no longer to his original (anatomic) fovea (Goldstein, 1927; Klüver, 1927). Such an enduring change in fixation, with a consequent change in the subjective middle, right, left, etc., in the visual field, has been interpreted as an indication of far-reaching plasticity in the relations between the visual field and its anatomic substrate.

Lateral Shift of Optical Axis

The most common form of persistent shift of the optical axis is a displacement of the midvertical meridian in the field. This displacement permits a hemianopic patient to see configurations of moderate size in their entirety, rather than split through the fixation point. As Fuchs has originally pointed out (1920, 1921, 1922), such readjustment of fixation is essentially identical with that seen in many strabismic eyes. The patient, instead of using his anatomic fovea, has adopted a new or vicarious fovea, which acts as the subjective center of the visual field.

The existence of such a pseudo-fovea is difficult to prove unless one pays attention to the position of some landmark, such as the normal blind spot in the field (Bender and Teuber, 1946, 1947b; Battersby, 1951; Feinberg, 1956). In 20 normal controls the blind spot was found to fall within its expected location, by our campimetric method, with an average error of less than ½°. In series A, however, 8 cases showed a definite and persistent displacement of the normal blind spot, away from its normal position. A characteristic example is the field in case A-28 (Figs. 38a,b), where the line dividing impaired and unimpaired parts of the field is shifted away from the midline, and with it the normal blind spot. We have already pointed out that such a shift in fixation will give the appearance of macular sparing for form as well as color.

Vertical Displacement of Optical Axis

Besides instances of lateral displacement of the midvertical meridian, one finds occasional instances of vertical displacement of the midhorizontal meridian. In such instances the patient avoids the obstruction of his central fixation, which results from an altitudinal defect, and the blind spot is correspondingly shifted upwards or downwards in the field. Such a downward shift can be quite marked in cases of inferior altitudinal hemianopia, as in our cases A-71 and A-102 (Figs. 5 and 6a,b).

Induced Ocular Torsion

Occasionally, massive field defects with irregular outline lead to fairly permanent torsions of the eye, so that the midvertical meridian appears tilted by several degrees against the true vertical. In routine perimetry, such deviations from the vertical are rarely recorded; however, an inspection of earlier fields obtained in gunshot wound cases (e.g., Poppelreuter, 1917, pp. 53–54, field 28–29) shows torsions of this sort, and we have seen persistent torsion in one case (Bn) in group SD.

Finally, markedly irregular scotomata in or near the macular region can induce strabismus and skew deviations of the eyes.

Visuospatial Organization in Cases of Pseudo-Fovea

From our results, eccentric fixation of a persistent sort evidently does accompany visual field defects. What is not known is how to interpret these phenomena. When the appearance of pseudo-foveae in hemianopics was first described in detail (Fuchs, 1920, 1922), the interpretation offered was somewhat teleologic: formation of a new or vicarious fovea was considered to indicate a plastic reorganization of the visual field, demonstrating considerable latitude in patterns of representation within the visual system. This plasticity was underscored by the further report by Fuchs that hemianopic patients exhibit heightened acuity in the area of their vicarious foveae. The new fovea had apparently assumed some of the functional characteristics of the old, indicating that acuity could become independent of the density of receptors, which is known to be maximal in the fovea. Our own results, however, obtained in earlier work with cases from group SD (Bender and Teuber, 1947b, 1948), are to some extent at variance with Fuchs' observations and interpretations (see also Sperry, 1945; Walls, 1951).

We found that even though eccentric fixation frequently occurs, it is not accompanied by any significant increase in acuity beyond the usually poor acuity of such eccentric regions. What is more surprising, the patients in group SD tended to exhibit persistent and sometimes serious errors in the estimation of distances, which seemed to be related to the existence of an abnormal reference point in their fields. Finally, it should be noted (as Goldstein has on several occasions, e.g., 1934, 1942) that in some of these cases the disturbances of perception associated with eccentric fixation go as far as to include a persistent or intermittent diplopia. Such diplopia is monocular, since it is present regardless of whether the patient uses the left eye, the right eye, or both. Monocular diplopia of this sort was particularly marked in cases of inferior altitudinal hemianopia; it was present in cases A-102 and A-140 as will be described below. The diplopia is analogous to that seen frequently for the squinted eye of patients with unilateral squint (see Bielschowsky, 1931). In both types of cases the monocular double images suggest the existence of a dual system of spatial reference: one organized around the anatomic fovea,

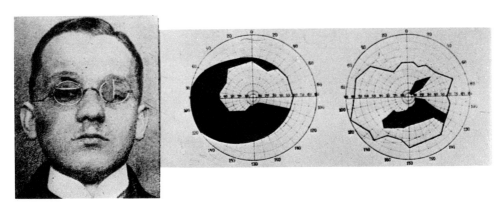

Figure 44. Hemianopic spectacles and their claimed effects on the binocular fields. On the left, Igersheimer's patient L with a spectacle frame carrying a horizontally oriented mirror before the right eye and a vertical mirror before the left. In the middle, the patient's binocular field as seen without the spectacles. On the right, binocular field plotted while patient wore hemianopic spectacles. Igersheimer reported that this patient adapted "within a few days" to this radical distortion of spatial organization of the visual field.

Reproduced by permission from J. Igersheimer, *Albrecht v. Graefes Arch. Ophthal.* 100:357–369 (1919).

the other around the false or vicarious fovea which is at some distance from the original one.

In a way, such persistently maladaptive functioning of the remnants of the visual field, in the presence of a shift in the visual axis, is rather surprising, especially if one considers recent reports on normal subjects wearing prismatic lenses or other distorting optical media in front of their eyes (Kohler, 1951). Such normal volunteers are said to accomplish a far-reaching reorganization of their visual fields, even beyond the extent reported originally by Stratton (1896, 1897). Patients with field defects apparently show less capacity than normal subjects to adapt themselves to disturbing factors in their fields of vision. The marked difficulty experienced by some patients may be analogous to other deficits in perceptual learning, such as the one demonstrated for the learning of a tactile discrimination after cerebral lesions (Ghent, Weinstein, Semmes, and Teuber, 1955).

In line with these considerations is the failure of our patients to benefit from hemianopic spectacles (e.g., Fig. 44; Igersheimer, 1919) whenever the attempt was made to improve their vision by such means. Thus, one of the patients wore prismatic lenses continuously for several days and repeated this three times. Every time, he complained that the prism, which transposed objects from the blind half of his field by 15° into the margin of the seeing half, disorganized his perception to the point of nausea. In contrast to similar experiences in normal subjects wearing such glasses, he was unable to adapt to the artificial change in visual stimulation.

The wearing of such glasses was originally suggested by Igersheimer (1919), who prescribed small mirrors mounted in spectacle frames. These spectacles were intended to direct light rays, which normally would have impinged on blind regions of the field, into seeing portions. Igersheimer considered these spectacles beneficial in several of his cases; he explicitly referred to Stratton's experiment (with inverting spectacles, 1896, 1897) as an analogous procedure; he believed that both his and Stratton's methods demonstrated a far-reaching plasticity of visuospatial organization in man. Several of Igersheimer's patients reported nearly complete adaptation to their spectacles within two days, so that the case for plasticity of projection would seem to be a strong one, particularly since some patients (e.g., Fig. 44) wore a vertically oriented mirror before one eye and a horizontal one before the other. The rapid acquisition of tolerance for such an asymmetric mode of visual stimulation seems to us to exceed anything subsequently achieved by Ivo Kohler and his subjects (1951).

Some doubts, however, are raised by Igersheimer's own account of persistent errors of visual localization whenever his patients were required to point at small luminous targets in the dark (Poppelreuter's pointing test, see Poppelreuter, 1917). These errors could still be demonstrated after habituation to the spectacles seemed complete in everyday visual surroundings (Igersheimer, 1919). These results would appear to be analogous to our observation that errors, for example, in the bisection of lines, persist in hemianopic patients with pseudo-foveae (Teuber and Bender, 1949).

It should finally be pointed out that we have as yet no clear evidence to explain why spontaneous adaptation of eccentric fixation (or pseudo-fovea) occurs in some instances and seems to be absent or only occasionally present in others. Nor is there sufficient information on the mode of origin of pseudo-foveae: whether the acquisition of a new fixation point is immediate or gradual, following the initial trauma. In either event, abnormalities of fixation after cerebral lesions underscore the limitations of available anatomic principles in predicting nature and extent of residual visual function.

7. Functioning versus Plotted Fields

FLUCTUATION, EXTINCTION, COMPLETION

In previous publications (Bender and Teuber, 1946, 1947a,b, 1949; Teuber and Bender, 1948a,b, 1949) we have stressed that routine perimetry results in fields which differ in a number of ways from the functioning field (see Gibson, 1950), i.e., the field experienced by the patient. Increased fluctuation of visual thresholds in amblyopic regions leads to obscuration or transient disappearance of visual objects. As a consequence of these fluctuations, the functioning field may be considerably smaller than the field which seems available on perimetric testing. The functioning field can be further reduced by an abnormal interaction of stimuli: objects that are seen in normal fashion when presented in isolation may become unreportable on intercurrent stimulation elsewhere in the field (extinction effect) (Fig. 45).

In contrast to fluctuation, obscuration, and extinction, which make the functioning field *smaller* than perimetry would indicate, there are mechanisms which occasionally *enlarge* the field beyond the area which one expects to function on the basis of perimetric records. Thus, visual configurations partly exposed to the unimpaired and partly to an amaurotic region of the field are often reported as complete (completion effect) (Fig. 46).

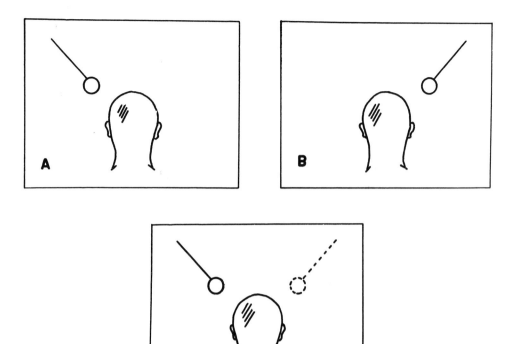

Figure 45. Extinction phenomenon shown schematically for a case of left occipito-parietal lesion. Single stimulation by a 5° target either in the left (A) or in the right (B) half of the field leads to prompt report on the patient's part. However, as soon as two targets are shown (C), one to the right, the other to the left, the patient reports that the one to the right "fades out," leaving only the one on the left visible. Analogous extinction of sensation on the right, on double simultaneous tactile stimulation of the right and left hands, also occurred in this case (SD-H). However, extinction can be limited to one sense modality.

Both extinction and completion effects, though under various names, have been described in numerous earlier reports (for extinction, see Loeb, 1884; Oppenheim, 1885; Bruns, 1886; Bender and Furlow, 1945a; Bender, 1952; for completion, see Poppelreuter, 1917; Fuchs, 1920; Goldstein, 1927; Bender and Teuber, 1946). We have added to these studies a special survey of a variant of completion, namely, the completion of apparent movement across scotomata which appear to be absolute on standard perimetry (Teuber and Bender, 1948c, 1950). In every case tested, patients experienced apparent motion across the area of the scotomata as soon as alternating lights appeared in fixed positions to either side of the area of blindness (see Fig. 47). The apparent motion effect was also obtained in case A-67 (see Figs. 16a,b), by placing the alternating lights to either side of the arc, which indicates that

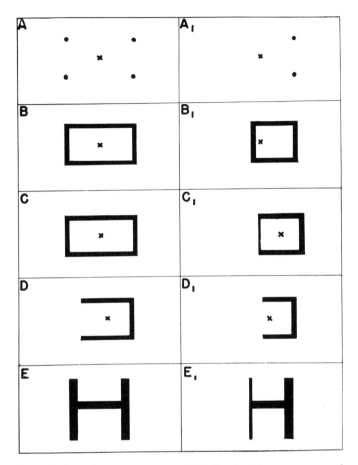

Figure 46. Completion phenomena, case SD-Bn (left homonymous hemianopia). On the left (A-E), patterns shown to patient by projection tachistoscope. The patient is seated at the opposite side of a translucent screen, where his fixation point is marked by X. Patterns A-C subtend 10° to either side of the fixation point along the horizontal meridian; D and E, 7° and 8°, respectively. The patient's reports of what he saw (first verbally, then by drawing) are given on the right side ($A_1 - E_1$). All these responses were obtained on $1/10$ sec. exposure. Frequent checks during testing showed that the patient did not react to single luminous targets in his blind (left) half-field. Nevertheless, some patterns were "completed" on tachistoscopy. Note that the patient did not complete the four-dot pattern (A_1) but reported only the two dots in his intact field. B_1 and C_1 were obtained with about equal frequency in response to pattern B (which was the same as C): the rectangle was reproduced nearly as a square, with a shorter portion to the left (B_1) or a thinner line to the left (C_1). When the rectangle was actually open towards the blind side, in pattern D, this particular patient did not complete it (see D_1). This suggests that the phenomenon was not simply a case of "closure" of incomplete figures. The last pattern (E) was promptly completed, but the patient insisted that the vertical line to the left was "less heavy."

Reproduced by permission from M. B. Bender and H.-L. Teuber, *Arch. Neurol. Psychiat.* 55:627–658 (1946).

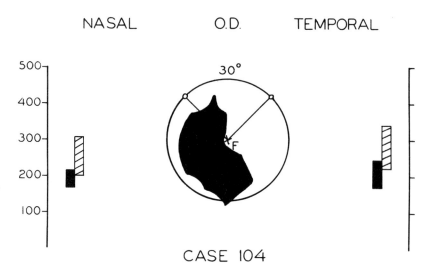

NASAL   O.D.   TEMPORAL

CASE 104

Figure 47. Diagram showing results of apparent motion experiments, involving motion across scotoma. The two radii extending from F (fixation point) to the 30° isopter indicate the placement of the intermittent lights. One light was always placed at F, the other at 30° from the fixation point. In one series of trials, this second light was placed in the right upper quadrant (at the point indicated by open circle). In another series of trials, the second light was placed at the corresponding point in the left upper quadrant. The ordinate, in milliseconds, gives the range of those time intervals (between alternate appearances of the two lights) for which apparent movement was reported by the patient. These time intervals are indicated for the patient by the black bar and for a normal control by the striped bar. Note that the patient reported apparent movement over a narrower range, and with more rapid rates of intermittence, than the normal control.

even complete separation of the stimuli by a scotoma did not interfere with the effect.

The importance of this phenomenon lies in its theoretic implications (see Wertheimer, 1912; Koffka, 1935; Köhler, 1940; Köhler and Wallach, 1944; Köhler and Held, 1949). Since apparent movement occurs in essentially normal fashion through amaurotic areas which are due to lesions in occipital structures, earlier psychophysiologic theories of apparent movement cannot be correct. These theories operated with the notion of an electrical process occurring in that portion of the visual cortex which lies between the areas to which the stimulus lights project. If such a theory were true, a traumatic lesion in cerebral structures lying between the two areas of projection should interfere with the perceptual phenomenon. The apparent motion obtained by our patients across scotomatous regions was so compelling that two of them believed such movement could be observed only because they had an area of blindness; they were unaware of the fact that the phenomenon in itself is normal.

AWARENESS OF SCOTOMA

Patient's Spontaneous Complaints

Often neglected as a source of data on visual disturbances after cerebral lesions are the patient's spontaneous complaints. Analysis of our material in this respect confirms the generalizations offered earlier, namely, that macular defects tend to be more obvious to the patient than peripheral defects, even though the latter may look much larger on perimetry.

In nearly all cases of homonymous defect, the patient complains that he has more difficulty with the eye contralateral to his occipital lesion; the homonymous nasal defect is frequently overlooked. As a result, the patient does not become aware of any impairment in the homolateral eye till after perimetric testing has shown him that both eyes are involved. We have already indicated our belief that these subjective phenomena are related to the physiologic and anatomic differences between nasal and temporal representation of the field, as originally described by Köllner (1914).

With few exceptions, the patients attribute their visual difficulties to some injury or disease of their eyes, at least until they are told about the connection between the cerebral lesion and the visual disturbance. In spite of such instructions, many patients continue to complain of foreign-body sensations in their eyes, and in some instances there is marked photophobia and excessive lacrimation; an extreme case was that of A-69. It is consistent with this observation that several of the patients who did not lose consciousness at the moment of injury asked the medical aid men to bandage their eyes, since they assumed that their eyes had been wounded, rather than the occipital region. Some patients related that this impression had been all the more vivid because they had seen startling phosphenes at the moment of impact, such as dazzling stars or whirls of light, either in white or in rainbow colors.

Predominance of Negative Scotomata

Only two cases in group A experienced positive scotomata; all the others (44 cases) referred to their scotomata as a blank or a void, i.e., their scotomata were negative. In each of the two exceptions (cases A-71 and A-99; Figs. 5 and 17a,b) there was an irregular field defect near the fixation point. In both instances, the patient complained of a faint "line" without definite shape or color which constantly transected objects they were inspecting.

In accordance with the usual negative character of the scotomata, a patient with pseudo-fovea is seldom aware of the fact that the optical axis has shifted. A particularly characteristic case is that of patient SD-B (Fig. 7a), who was completely unaware of the fact that he was not looking directly at objects; instead he insisted that his gaze was normally oriented, but complained that objects below the fixation point appeared indistinct.

Entoptic Visibility of Scotomata on Special Testing

It is a puzzling fact that under special conditions some patients can be made aware of a scotoma by protracted testing. Thus, prolonged inspection of a brightly illuminated white surface can make part or all of a scotoma visible as a dark cloud; inspection of a colored surface occasionally produces an entoptic image of a scotoma in complementary colors (such as the claw in the left upper macular quadrant in case A-99; Figs. 17a,b). Such strange effects have been reported previously by Brückner (1917). If a patient develops a complementary after-image in the "seeing" portions of his field, after the colored stimulus surface has been withdrawn, the after-image encloses an ill-defined area corresponding to the scotoma, and this enclosed area now appears in the original color of the stimulus surface. These phenomena are difficult to explain on the basis of known physiology and anatomy of the visual system. Similar problems are raised by the frequent occurrence of ordinary completion in after-images which extend into areas of scotoma (see Fuchs, 1921; Bender and Teuber, 1947a; Hebel and Luther, 1947; Bender and Kahn, 1949). It is for this reason that after-imagery cannot be used as a short cut to perimetric testing of defective fields, as has at times been suggested (Vujić and Levi, 1939).

Absence of Anton Syndrome (Denial of Blindness)

In 7 of our cases the acute injury by gunshot wound produced an initial period of apparent total blindness lasting for hours or days. In this phase the symptoms resembled those seen after bilateral thrombosis of branches of the posterior cerebral arteries in patients with cerebrovascular disease (Symonds and Mackenzie, 1957). However, in contrast to many of the latter cases, the patient with a gunshot wound is keenly aware of the fact that he has been blinded. Several of our case histories include reports of violent, if appropriate, reactions on the patient's part; for example, he implores the medical aid man to shoot him on the field, since he does not want to survive in the presence of total blindness. This behavior contrasts of course with the clinically well-known denial of blindness (Anton syndrome: Anton, 1898; Redlich and Bonvicini, 1908; Redlich and Dorsey, 1945), seen occasionally in bilateral occipital involvement following conditions other than acute trauma. The reason for this difference in reaction to cortical blindness may be a difference in the general condition of the central nervous system; conceivably denial of blindness requires diffuse and widespread cerebral lesions, in addition to those involving the higher visual pathways themselves.

The Problem of Total Blindness after
Destruction of the Geniculostriate System

Since there was no permanent blindness in any patient in groups A and SD, we cannot confirm or deny the common belief (e.g., Marquis, 1935) that total destruction of the human geniculostriate system should lead to complete and permanent blindness; this would be in marked contrast to the effect of complete ablation of striate cortex in subhuman primates, which is followed by the return of some primitive light perception, consisting in global reactions to luminous flux, as shown by Klüver (1942a). There have been repeated attempts (e.g., by Monakow, 1914, and by Marquis, 1935) to arrange earlier observations on subhuman forms (e.g., Panizza, 1855; Munk, 1881), together with clinical observations on man, into a phylogenetic series. According to these views, the higher the phyletic status of the organism, the more dependent vision becomes upon the integrity of cortex.

The proof for such increasing corticalization of vision runs into difficulties, since tests of residual visual capacities in man and lower animals can rarely be compared (Teuber, 1955; Weiskrantz, 1958). In monkeys with partial destruction of the striate cortex, surprisingly few residual visual deficits can be demonstrated after the first two weeks following operation (see Klüver, 1937, 1941; Settlage, 1939a,b; Harlow, 1939). In man, the residual part of the field continues to exhibit subtle but significant abnormalities (see below), a finding which might reflect either a genuine difference between the visual systems of man and subhuman primate, or, again, a difference in the sensitivity of visual tests that can be applied to either species.

Even more puzzling is the supposed absence of all light perception following complete loss of striate cortex in man. Marie and Chatelin (1915), who in World War I examined nearly as many cases of gunshot wound of the visual pathways as are reviewed in our present report, did not encounter anything but *transient* blindness, a finding consistent with our own. In fact, in the two cases of initial blindness which are reported in some detail by Marie and Chatelin (1915), the blindness had already been replaced by "vague impressions of luminosity," by the time the patients came under their care. In both instances, distinct vision returned eventually, despite extensive bilateral destruction of the occipital lobes, and in both this recovery was reported to have begun with the central part of the field. Wilbrand and Saenger (1918), basing their studies on several hundred cases seen by themselves and others, declared categorically that no single case of permanent blindness (after lesions of the suprachiasmal visual system) had come to their attention. All 5 of the cases which they were able to find in the literature seemed unconvincing for either or both of two reasons: insufficient length of the survival period following the trauma or inadequate testing.

Testing in man should certainly include a search for residual light perception after prolonged dark adaptation (see Klüver, 1927; Bender and Teuber, 1949; Krieger and Bender, 1951), particularly since Klüver has demonstrated reactions to light under such conditions in monkeys after bilateral occipital lobectomy. As far as we can ascertain, no tests of this sort have been applied in cases of supposedly lasting blindness, such as that reported by Morax, Moreau, and Castelain (1919). Among 86 patients with field defects resulting from gunshot wounds of the central visual pathways, this was the only one who reputedly showed permanent and total blindness in the entire visual field. By contrast, loss of vision after bilateral infarction of occipital lobes (in vascular disease) is said to produce "lasting blindness" in one quarter of all cases (Symonds and Mackenzie, 1957). Here, again, tests under conditions of dark adaptation would be of interest.

The Density of Scotomata: Relative or Absolute?

Similar doubts have arisen with regard to the nature of regional blindness; Poppelreuter (1917), for one, has claimed that no scotoma after penetrating lesions of central visual pathways could ever be "absolute," i.e., completely lacking in light perception. In all instances of partial blindness, he reported, areas of apparent loss of vision could be shown to possess residual function; this could be done simply by increasing either the size or the luminous intensity of the test object. For Poppelreuter, scotomata were thus areas of increased difficulty of seeing, rather than islands of blindness. In a similar way paralysis after lesions of the motor cortex has been considered, not as a sign of absence of movement, but as a sign of increased difficulty in eliciting movements (Franz and Oden, 1917; Franz, 1923) or a change in the "adequate stimulus for motion" (Walshe, 1947, 1954; Clark, 1948; Denny-Brown and Botterell, 1948; Denny-Brown, 1951).

Available evidence unfortunately is insufficient to settle this issue. If complete destruction of all of the striate cortex is compatible with some return of global light perception, partial destruction leading to regional scotomata might likewise be associated with diminution rather than complete abolition of vision. One might even go further, and assume that lesions below a critical size in the visual cortex might fail to produce demonstrable scotomata (Weiskrantz, 1958). It is just as possible, however, that complete destruction of the cortical substrate in both occipital lobes is a prerequisite for the appearance of some primitive light perception, if such light perception should return at all.

Our own data suggest in any event that some scotomata and some seemingly blind half-fields in cases of homonymous hemianopia are capable of mediating reactions to light. Thus, it was noted during flicker perimetry (Battersby, 1951) that for 5 out of 10 hemianopic patients, fusion thresholds (though greatly raised) could be obtained in areas which had seemed totally blind on standard perimetry. Similarly, in tests of dark adaptation, all 5 patients were able to discriminate the presence from the absence of a light directed at seemingly blind regions in their field, after dark adaptation had continued for more than 30 minutes. The difficulty with interpreting such evidence, however, is the obvious one: in some cases at least, the stimulus intensity has to be raised to such levels that diffusion of light through the media of the eye (into the seeing portion) becomes unavoidable. Such data are therefore as inconclusive as were Poppelreuter's in 1917.

Our own earlier studies of completion phenomena likewise suggest that there are degrees of blindness, so to speak, in hemianopic or scotomatous regions. We observed, first, that completion was not obligatory, for it occurred in some but not all cases of field defect; secondly, completion—where it did occur—could often be shown to be due to some residual function (Bender and Teuber, 1946, 1947b); lastly, there were cases analogous to the classic ones, in which completion seemed identical with the normal phenomenon of closure of incomplete figures. In these cases the part of the figure which fell into the blind region of the field could be omitted without upsetting the patient's report that he had seen a whole figure.

The observations on the completion of apparent movement across scotomata should be similarly interpreted. These data indicate that perception can be spatially continuous even though the stimuli are exposed to either side of a discontinuity in the neural substrate. This phenomenon is distinct from that of residual light perception in the intervening region itself: when one or the other of the stimulus lights was manipulated so that it fell into the region of the scotoma, the apparent movement effect was immediately abolished and the patient reported merely a single flickering light in the area corresponding to that target which had remained outside the area of blindness in an adjacent portion of the visual field.

Relative Vulnerability of Different Aspects of Vision

The Sequence of Reappearance of Functions in the Field of Vision

Cases of initial total blindness following gunshot wounds of the posterior lobes of the brain are particularly revealing if one observes the gradual recovery of visual functions. As pointed out by Poppelreuter (1917) and others (Lhermitte and Ajuriaguerra, 1942), recovery takes place in definite stages, by which different aspects of vision return in a regular sequence: first to recover is an undifferentiated sensation of light, without shape, color, or orientation in space. After that, movement of a light may be distinguished from a stationary light, but the patient is still unable to indicate the direction or speed of the movement. Orientation of objects in visual space becomes possible at about the time when vague and "fuzzy" contours are reported. Still later, color experiences may return, often after a period of intense red coloration of the entire field (erythropsia). Published reports indicate even a fairly definite sequence with regard to the recovery of different colors (Lhermitte and Ajuriaguerra, 1942), but we have no data of our own on this subject.

Degrees of Deficit in Different Regions of Permanently Defective Fields

It is of considerable theoretical interest that the gradation of visual defects surrounding absolute scotomata (in fields in which the defects have

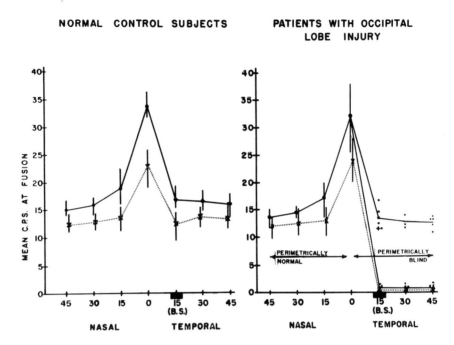

Figure 48. Fusion thresholds for flickering light for 10 normal controls (graph on left) and 10 patients with homonymous hemianopiae resulting from penetrating wounds involving the occipital lobes (graph on right). Vertical bars indicate range of fusion thresholds. In the hemianopic group, the eye tested was always the one in which the blind half-field was in the temporal region. Tests in this region revealed that 5 patients could perceive and roughly localize the flickering light (2° target) within the blind areas, while the other 5 could not. Note the slight but significant drop of fusion thresholds taken in the area of the normal blind spot (BS), in the curves for the normal group, indicating that the subject reacts to scattered light. The fusion thresholds in the seemingly intact half-fields for the hemianopic patients were slightly but significantly reduced as compared with corresponding control values. Solid curves based on 2° target, dotted curves on ½° target.

become permanent) duplicates the order in which functions reappear during recovery following acute injury. Thus, the minimal amount of vision possible in a scotomatous region is the perception of unlocalizable, shapeless, and colorless light. Surrounding such areas one often finds, on careful testing, an intermediate zone in which orientation is possible but poor, and in which colors are faded and contours fuzzy. Still further away from the area of maximal involvement, localization is adequate and contours and colors fairly well defined.

As Lashley (1930) has stressed, such sequences indicate that the strict topographic mapping of the visual field onto the striate cortex does not extend to what might be called levels of visual function. There is a functional hierarchy of different aspects of vision which can be derived from their relative vulnerability to cerebral lesions.

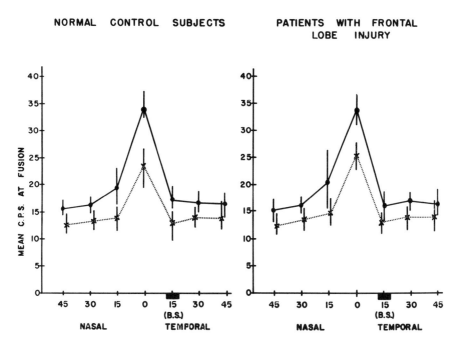

Figure 49. Fusion thresholds for flickering light for 10 normal control subjects (graph on left) and 10 patients with frontal lobe injury (graph on right). There is no significant difference between values for controls and for patients with frontal lobe injury. For further details, see legend to Figure 48.

Special Role of Flicker Perimetry in Demonstrating Minimal Losses and Minimal Remnants of Function

During the first World War, Riddoch (1917) pointed out that perimetry with moving targets often shows fields that are markedly wider than those obtained with stationary targets alone. His method has been generally accepted in clinical practice. Where facilities are available, a somewhat more precise addition to the methods of field-taking can be provided in the form of flicker perimetry (see Phillips, 1933; Teuber and Bender, 1948a, 1949; Teuber, 1950; Battersby, 1951). This method can reveal both minimal losses in seemingly intact areas of the field of vision and minimal remnants of vision in areas which appear to be totally amaurotic on perimetry. Thus, a special study (Battersby, 1951) of 10 of our cases in group A by flicker perimetry (as described above) showed that, in all instances of field defect, fusion thresholds of flicker were reduced in seemingly intact portions of the field. The depression of thresholds was maximal near a scotoma and less marked as the area tested was further away from the region of obvious impairment (see Fig. 48). On the other hand, half of the hemianopic patients perceived a flickering light when the light was directed into the seemingly blind regions of their fields. Since this did not appear in all hemianopics, it seems unlikely that these patients merely reacted to stray light entering the less impaired portions of their fields (see Battersby, 1951).

In flicker perimetry (as described in our section on methods), fusion thresholds are determined for different positions in the visual field. In this respect the method differs from exposures of flickering light to the central field alone, without attempts at defining differences in the response of selected retinal regions (see Klüver, 1942a; Christian and Schmitz, 1942; Halstead, 1947). Such a use of flickering light, directed at the central region of the field, also shows abnormalities in response, in the form of reductions in fusion thresholds. Thus, men with gunshot wounds of the occipital region show abnormally low fusion rates for rotating black and white patterns (Masson discs, see Christian and Schmitz, 1942; Bender and Teuber, 1948, 1949; or logarithmic spirals, see Bender and Teuber, 1947b, 1948, 1949). Similarly, Klüver's classic study of residual vision in monkeys with bilateral occipital lobectomies (1942a) showed that for such animals an intermittent light, flickering at 1 per sec., was indistinguishable from a steady light of half intensity.

In 1947 Halstead reported maximal reduction in fusion thresholds (for a centrally fixated light source) in patients with frontal lobe resections for removal of neoplasms; no reduction was found by him in patients with corresponding occipital lobe resections. In contrast with this report for cases of neoplastic disease of the brain, we did not find such reduction of fusion thresholds after frontal lesions in our gunshot wound cases, either in group SD (see Bender and Teuber, 1947, 1948; Teuber and Bender, 1949) or in group A (see Fig. 49; and Battersby, 1951; Battersby, Bender, and Teuber, 1951). In both groups (A and SD) there was reduction of fusion thresholds after occipital injury, but no reduction (in fact a slight but insignificant elevation of fusion thresholds) in men with frontal penetration (see also Teuber, 1952).

Recently, measurements of this type have been extended to cases of neoplastic disease of the brain, with analogous results (Battersby and Bender, 1958). Of special interest is the demonstration that appropriate choice of stimulus parameters will reveal significant losses in CFF in the foveal region, in cases where the perimetric defects appear to be restricted to the periphery of the field. Moreover, a recent application of the two-flash technique (Battersby and Wagman, 1959) suggests that the reduction of CFF in defective fields is attributable to an abnormal interaction of stimuli successively applied. Thus, if a conditioning flash is presented to a patient, and followed within a critical time by a test flash, the threshold for the first flash may be normal, but that for the second flash greatly raised, indicating a characteristic abnormality in recovery of the visual system from the effects of the first flash.

Dark Adaptation

Results of measuring dark adaptation were analogous. Using Wald's modification (1941) of the Hecht-Shlaer adaptometer (1938), Krieger and

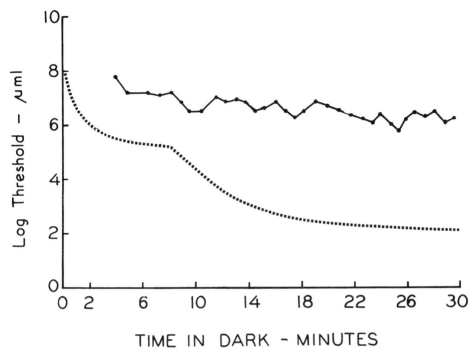

TIME IN DARK - MINUTES

Figure 50. Dark adaptation curve (solid line) for a patient with bilateral hemi-anopia and peephole vision (case A-29, see Figs. 13a,b). For comparison, a dark adaptation curve has been plotted for a normal subject. Note that the patient's curve fails to descend as far as the control curve, and that it lacks the normal break between the earlier "cone" section and the subsequent "rod" section.

Bender demonstrated (Krieger and Bender, 1949, 1951; Krieger, 1952) a marked slowing in the adaptation curve obtained for parts of the field that seemed intact on ordinary perimetry. In addition, these dark adaptation curves showed markedly increased variability, and a failure to reach the same levels of ultimate sensitivity as the corresponding regions of normal fields. Similar results (though limited to foveal vision) had been obtained earlier (Behr, 1931; Ullrich, 1943; Ruesch, 1944; Christian and Umbach, 1947); these had been interpreted as an indication for the existence of central factors in the dark adaptation process (see Behr, 1931). Of particular interest is the shape of the dark adaptation curve for A-29, the case of maximal con-centric contraction of the field (Fig. 50). This patient's vision was restricted to a "peephole" in the center of the field (see Figs. 13a,b). Dark adaptation in this remnant of the visual field was grossly abnormal: over a 30-minute period, the curve descended only very slightly, indicating little gain in sensi-tivity with time; the variability was greater than in normal controls, and there was no sign of the secondary inflection which appears in normal dark adap-tation curves at the point where cone adaptation is assumed to be completed (see Fig. 50, normal control curve).

Diffuseness of Minimal Losses

The fact that fusion thresholds for flickering light (and absolute thresholds in dim light) were reduced in areas far removed from any obvious scotoma is a special instance of dissociation of functions (Riddoch, 1917) in different zones of an impaired field. All the hemianopics tested showed reduced fusion thresholds of flicker and impaired dark adaptation throughout the seemingly normal half of the field of vision. This observation is in marked contrast to the reports for other species, such as Lashley's statement (1939) that rats with small remnants of the field of vision (only 700 nondegenerated cells in one lateral geniculate body) have perfectly unimpaired visual functions. On the basis of his experiments, Lashley concluded that areas of visual cortex within 1 to 2 mm. from the margin of a lesion produced by cortical ablation can function normally. Since this is not true for man, it is important to point out that the apparent integrity of visual functions in the rat may be due to the limited number of visual tests that can be employed in such a species.

The diffuse impairment in vision in the presence of seemingly focal lesions in man is all the more paradoxical, if one accepts the belief that secondary (degenerative) changes in visual cortex should be limited to the immediate vicinity of the lesion. The usual histologic methods seem to suggest that degeneration in the cortex, around a small lesion (in rodent, carnivore, and, possibly, primate) does not extend for more than 1 to 2 mm. beyond the margin of the lesion (see, e.g., LeGros Clark, 1941). These findings need to be reassessed with the use of different histologic methods, such as modified Bielschowsky stains (see Glees and Nauta, 1955). Use of these techniques suggests a much wider spread of degeneration of terminals (at least for the rodent), possibly crossing the midline from one striate cortex to the other (see Nauta and van Straaten, 1947; Nauta, 1950; Nauta and Bucher, 1954). Recent electrophysiologic studies have led to the claim of diffuse bilateral distribution of evoked potentials in cat's visual cortex on focal retinal stimulation by light (Doty, 1958).

General Association and Dissociation of Visual Symptoms

Areas of the visual field in which flicker perception and dark adaptation are depressed invariably show other subtle but systematic visual alterations. Thus, color discrimination for small targets is slightly impaired, and thresholds for apparent and real motion are altered (see Teuber and Bender, 1948c, 1949). A case in point is furnished by A-48 (Figs. 36a,b); here the patient's hemiachromatopia was most conspicuous as a color defect, but also involved fusion thresholds of flicker (which were depressed, see Fig. 42), as well as other visual functions.

It is important to realize that the original description by Riddoch of a "dissociation" of visual functions in defective fields is easily misinterpreted to mean a separate cerebral localization for different "moieties" of vision (Hines, 1942). Actually, the evidence first brought forward by Riddoch, and since then amply confirmed, indicates that there is an order of fragility for visual functions, rather than a separate localization. To prove the latter, one not only needs evidence that some aspects of the visual function are more readily impaired than others, but must demonstrate the presence of double dissociation, by means of which perception of form or motion would be selectively lost or preserved. This, however, is precisely what does not happen. Perception of motion may remain when perception of form has become impaired, but the reverse does not occur, that is, one does not find intact perception of form in areas impaired for the visual perception of motion (Teuber, 1960).

Far more radical claims for dissociation have been made. Various "elementary" aspects of visual performance, such as perception of color, form, or motion, are considered dissociable, as a group, from appropriate reactions to the spatial position or to the meaning of visually presented objects. Concepts of visuospatial agnosia and visual object agnosia imply such a selective impairment of function on "higher," or gnostic, levels while visuosensory functions continue to be intact. If these selective losses could be demonstrated as readily as the everyday clinical usage of "agnosia" would seem to suggest, one would have to accept a separate localization for "lower" and "higher" aspects of vision. Traditionally, such a separation has been claimed to exist with elementary functions represented in the striate cortex ("visuosensory" area), and complex gnostic functions in the surrounding cortex of the occipital lobe ("visuopsychic" regions). Evidence for such a separation of functions is far from compelling, either on the behavioral or anatomic level; the commonly accepted syndromes of agnosia, for visual space or for visual objects, require careful scrutiny.

Visuospatial agnosia. In earlier reports based on selected cases from group SD, we have described concomitant changes in perception of size, depth, and motion (Bender and Teuber, 1947b, 1948). These alterations in perception were maximal in homonymous half-fields, quadrants, or even sectors of the visual field. In these areas, visual objects appeared to be abnormally far away, their contours faded, and their apparent size reduced, as compared with less impaired regions of the field. These patients did not show any disturbances in the localization of objects when vision was excluded. Nevertheless, we do not believe these systematic distortions of visual space should be designated as visuospatial agnosia, since such a term would imply that the impairment is selective for the spatial organization of objects. Instead, areas with maximal change in spatial organization also exhibited maximal impairment in the resolution of flickering light (i.e., reduced CFF), showing that the disturbance was not restricted to the spatial order of visual stimuli. Similar alterations in vision were found among the late after-effects of gunshot wounds involving the posterior lobe substance (group A). As we shall see, however, visuospatial disorders which had been continuous in group SD were only episodic in those patients of group A who showed such alterations.

The mode of onset of visuospatial disorders in group SD is not fully known, but some of our data indicate that change in relative localization of visual objects could appear as an instantaneous effect of the impact of the missile. Thus, one of the men sustained a penetrating wound of the right occipital region; he was only momentarily stunned, climbed out of his armored vehicle, and attempted to run for cover. He immediately noticed that objects on his left side had become invisible; he had acquired a left homonymous hemianopia. Everything on his right, however, seemed curiously tilted. He therefore adjusted his posture to the apparent slope of the ground, with the result that he stumbled and fell when he tried to run. Another patient reported that immediately after his wounding, objects looked as if surrounded by fuzzy fringes; they had become very small and seemed abnormally distant; this again was maximal for certain regions of the visual field. It is clear that all these subjective distortions in the visual field involve relative localization (see Holmes, 1945); the resulting errors of localization are thus quite different from the erratic performance found in cases of disorientation which, in our series at least, did not appear as a selectively visual disturbance.

These systematic distortions in the coordinates of visual space should be distinguished from more general disorders of orientation which are sometimes described as characteristic of men with severe injury to occipital or occipito-parietal structures (Lange, 1936; see also Paterson and Zangwill, 1944a,b; Zangwill, 1951; Faust, 1955). Experimental analyses of these disorders of orientation in a large number of patients from group A has shown that (a) these more general disorders of orientation (route-finding) are independent of the presence or absence of field defect; (b) they occur particularly often with parietal lesions (of either hemisphere or both); and (c) they should not be designated as a visual agnosia, since the difficulty in route-finding exists independently of whether or not the patient uses vision or other sense modalities, such as touch and kinesthesis (Semmes, Weinstein, Ghent, and Teuber, 1955; Weinstein, Semmes, Ghent, and Teuber, 1956; see also Bay, 1954).

Visual object agnosia. The most far-reaching claims for dissociation of levels of visual function are implied in the concept of visual object agnosia. According to the classic definition of this term (Freud, 1891), a patient should show severe disturbances in the recognition of objects by sight, and this in the absence of dementia or elementary visual disturbances sufficient to account for the gnostic defect.

We have not encountered in either group A or group SD such dissociation of "higher" from "lower" aspects of visual function. An abnormal slowness in the recognition of objects by sight was found occasionally in the first month following gunshot wound of the posterior third of the brain, but this

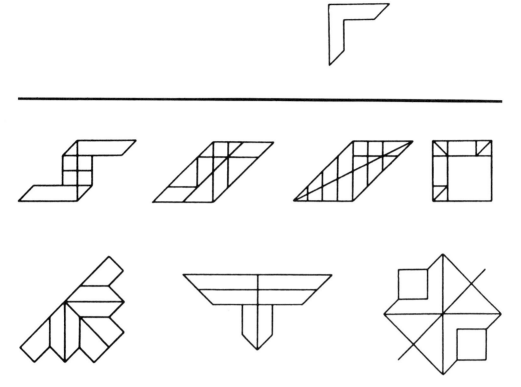

Figure 51. Sample page of Gottschaldt test. The subject is required to find the figure at the top within each of the lower (embedding) figures, and to trace it completely with pencil within each of the embedding figures.

Reproduced by permission from H.-L. Teuber and S. Weinstein, *Arch. Neurol. Psychiat.* 76:309–379 (1956).

impairment existed on all levels, since there were, associated with the seemingly gnostic defect, various additional alterations, such as abnormal fluctuations of thresholds, and difficulties with spatial as well as temporal discriminations.

It is true that group A patients with field defects continued to show slowness of recognition on the tachistoscope, as well as persistent difficulties in the visual searching for objects (Teuber, Battersby, and Bender, 1949, 1951). However, such residual difficulties could also be found in men with cerebral lesions outside the higher visual pathways (Teuber and Bender, 1951; Teuber and Weinstein, 1956). We do not believe that such residual symptoms merit the label of visual object agnosia.

Similarly, men with occipital lesions continue to show marked impairment in the perception of hidden figures (Fig. 51) analogous to those constructed by Gottschaldt (1926, 1929); this impairment can still be demonstrated ten years after the wounding. However, a detailed study of this deficit in group A (Teuber and Weinstein, 1956) revealed that men with wounds of entrance into any lobe—occipital, temporal, parietal, or frontal, in either hemisphere or both—showed about equal degrees of impairment on such hidden figure tasks (Fig. 52). The impairment was clearly independent of the presence or absence of visual field defects. Only men with aphasia showed selectively greater impairment than the rest of the brain-injured population, who in turn fell significantly below the performance level of the control group with peripheral nerve injuries (see Fig. 53). Essentially parallel results were obtained more recently for figures with reversible or ambiguous perspective (see Rubin, 1915; Cohen, 1959). Whatever the interpretation of such abnormal reaction to hidden or reversible figures should be, the abnormality cannot be equated with agnosia in the usual sense of this term.

Similarly, we have not encountered any case of isolated dyslexia in either group SD or group A; wherever disturbances of reading were marked, there was noticeable aphasia. The dyslexia thus appeared merely as one aspect of a more general disturbance of language.

We should stress that even in cases of peephole vision, such as A-29, the patient failed to show any genuine signs of agnosia or alexia. The patient with the small remnant of central vision actually worked steadily as a mail sorter; he took each letter, carefully pulled the address across the small area of macular sparing in his visual field, and then threw the letter (without looking) into the appropriate receptacle on the shelf provided for sorting. This performance is all the more remarkable if one considers the usual anatomic interpretation of gnostic deficits: the primary visual receiving area, i.e., the striate cortex, is thought to mediate elementary visual sensation; impulses are conducted from this primary zone to a surrounding "visuopsychic," or "associative" region, usually homologized with Brodmann's areas 18 and 19 in the occipital lobe.

The cyto-architectonic status of these prestriate subdivisions is a dubious one; both can be distinguished unequivocally from area 17 with its characteristic stripe of Gennari, but the differences between 18 and 19, or between 19 and surrounding parietal and temporal cortex, are gradual, and the criteria offered for their distinction ambiguous (Lashley and Clark, 1946). Isolation of the striate cortex from these prestriate regions either by transection or destruction of the latter is apparently not followed by agnosia-like symptoms in animals, and there is no convincing evidence that it should be so followed in man (see Lashley, 1942, 1948; Evarts, 1952). In cases like that of A-29, the central visual field is certainly isolated from surrounding structures, at least on the cerebral surface, if our conceptions of retinotopical projection are at all valid. Nevertheless, no true agnosia was found in this case, or in similar traumatic conditions. It is perhaps significant that in those clinical cases where agnosia

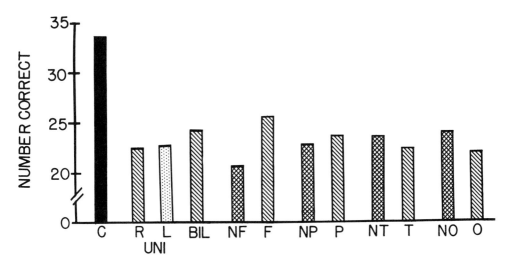

Figure 52. Mean number of figures correctly traced by controls (C) and brain-injured subjects grouped according to location of lesion. R, right unilateral lesion; L, left unilateral lesion; BIL, bilateral lesion; F, P, T, and O, indicate frontal, parietal, temporal, and occipital, respectively; NF, NP, NT, and NO indicate nonfrontal, nonparietal, etc.

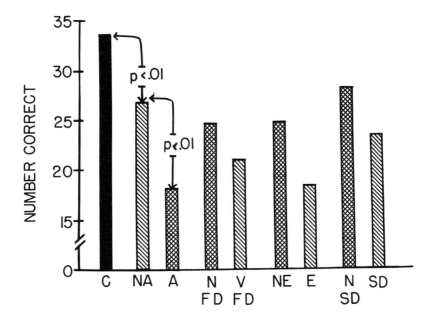

Figure 53. Mean number of figures traced correctly by controls (C), and by brain-injured subjects grouped according to presence or absence of aphasia (A), visual field defect (VFD), epilepsy (E), and somatosensory defect (SD). Absence of a given defect is indicated by N.

Reproduced by permission from Teuber and Weinstein, *loc. cit.*

has been claimed to exist, the visual fields either had not been reported or could not be obtained; the disturbance characteristically resulted from a diffuse vascular process or a toxic condition such as severe carbon monoxide poisoning (see Adler, 1941, 1950).

If we accept the classic definition of agnosia, we must say that not a single instance of this disorder has been seen among our cases of gunshot wound, or among those of Marie and Chatelin (1915), or of Wilbrand and Saenger (1918). This could mean either that object agnosia in the classic sense does not exist (Bay, 1950), or that the condition requires a lesion which is rarely or never seen after penetrating missile wounds. Thus, bilateral lesions of the posterior (basal) temporal lobes might be necessary (Milner, 1958), but a penetrating wound that produces such a lesion is incompatible with survival. It should be noted, however, that as methods of testing become more accurate, reports of agnosia become less and less numerous, while controversies regarding the earlier published cases increase.

The bilateral temporal lobe syndrome. To be sure, bilateral temporal lobe lesions in the monkey are said to result in agnosia-like difficulties with visual discrimination learning (Klüver and Bucy, 1938, 1939; Blum, Chow and Pribram, 1950; Chow, 1952a,b; Riopelle et al., 1953; Mishkin, 1954; Mishkin and Pribram, 1954; Mishkin and Hall, 1955). [These changes are definitely not found after destruction of prestriate regions (Lashley, 1948; Evarts, 1952).] However, there are serious questions about the nature of the alteration in the animal's behavior (see Teuber, 1955): Is the defect really specific for *visual* discrimination, as claimed? More recent observations cast doubt on this assumption (Santibañez and Pinto, 1957; Pasik, Pasik, Battersby, and Bender, 1958a,b), although there is some experimental evidence that favors it (Ettlinger, 1959; Pribram and Barry, 1956; Weiskrantz and Mishkin, 1958; Wilson, 1957; Wilson and Mishkin, 1959). Moreover, there is the possibility that the discriminatory difficulties reflect some subtle alteration in elementary visual function, such as abnormal fluctuation of thresholds, which then leads to disintegration of perceptual patterns or interference with the control of voluntary gaze. Both types of disturbance have been described for man: the fragmentation of images by Faust (1947a,b; see also Wolpert, 1924) and the ataxia or outright paralysis of gaze by Balint, as early as 1909. Neither of these conditions should be subsumed under the traditional concept of agnosia, which requires a modality-specific loss in recognition of objects in the presence of essentially normal sensorimotor function. Perhaps it is wiser to avoid the term "agnosia" altogether and to specify instead various degrees of difficulty in recognition, without reference to their etiology. For analogous reasons, "apraxia" (Liepmann, 1900, 1905, 1906) seems to us a dangerous term. Whoever claims the existence of visual agnosia, apraxia, or pure dyslexia (see Jung, 1948), should assume, it seems to us, the burden of empirical proof (Semmes, 1953; Teuber, 1955). Such proof entails the most thorough analysis of visual performance on "sensory" as well as "higher," or cognitive, levels. Even more difficult to establish are the recurrent claims of loss in visualization or other changes in imagery (see Charcot, 1883) following occipital injury or disease.

PERSISTENCE OF PLOTTED RESIDUAL DEFECTS AND
ROLE OF PAROXYSMAL ALTERATIONS

Episodic Alterations in Visual Fields

It is generally agreed that field defects found a year after penetrating lesions of the posterior lobe substance will persist indefinitely. Our own material corroborates this general assumption, since in all instances in group A, field defects had been present for at least 5 years and persisted without change for another 5 to 7 years. Of particular interest is the case of patient A-71 (Fig. 5), whose inferior altitudinal hemianopia was the result of a gutter-type gunshot wound sustained in September, 1918. His field defects had been plotted in various clinics, at approximately yearly intervals since 1920, and were plotted by us on three different occasions from 1949 to 1957. The fields showed no change over the entire period of 37 years.

This same patient has experienced occasional episodes of a migrainous character, during which he localized "flames" and "stars" in the blind area of his field. At such times the area of blindness increased, leaving him temporarily with complete amaurosis. These attacks have recurred irregularly, several times a year, throughout the 39 years that have elapsed since he was injured. The case thus illustrates extreme persistence of field defects, together with recurrent exacerbations, akin to migraine attacks or scintillating scotomata. Such episodic changes in the state of a defective field of vision are actually not uncommon (see Poppelreuter, 1917; Russell and Whitty, 1955); since they are transient, they do not detract from the chronic and unvarying character of the field defects themselves.

The paroxysmal alterations in vision were recorded in 15 cases in group A (the group consisting of 232 men with gunshot wounds of the brain). Of these 15 men, 12 had permanent visual field defects and were thus included among the 46 whose condition is described in this report. Three additional men with visual attacks had occipito-temporal lesions without demonstrable field defects.

In their simplest form, such visual attacks were episodes altogether restricted to the visual modality (8 of the 15 cases). In the other instances, the visual symptoms represented the first stage of a sequence (within a single episode) leading from visual to sensory Jacksonian attacks or frank convulsions. Following such an episode, there often was an increase in the blind area of the field, lasting from a few minutes to several days.

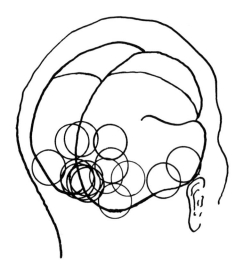

Figure 54. Composite diagram showing distribution of bone defects in 15 cases with recurrent "visual attacks," as defined in text. The bone defects are schematized by placing a circle around the center of each defect (without attempting to account for size, shape, or depth of lesions). Note the preponderance of lesions on the right side of the brain.

An example of long-lasting exacerbation of symptoms after each episode is furnished by case A-161. This man was struck by a shell fragment in the right occipital protuberance; the wound caused a left homonymous hemianopia, but this decreased until only small paracentral scotomata remained. During his visual attacks, the patient sees a vertical bar, dazzling in all colors —red, white and blue, "like a rotating barber pole." At the same time everything else in the field of vision becomes blank "like an empty screen." Such an episode lasts a few minutes but is followed invariably by a period of complete left homonymous hemianopia, lasting from one and a half to two days.

A remarkable feature of these visual episodes is their association with injuries of a fairly restricted region of the brain. If we limit this survey to the 15 cases in which the visual component was the earliest (and often, the only) sign of an attack, we obtain a distribution of wounds of entrance as shown in Figure 54. It is apparent that most of the lesions are clustered about the occiput; only two lesions are found farther forward in the temporal lobe. Moreover, one notes that the right hemisphere is implicated in 13 of the 15 cases, a curious disproportion.

The predominant association between right hemisphere lesions and visual aurae in our group is perhaps not an isolated occurrence, since similar relationships appear in two other studies. In their survey of hallucinations in neurologic disease, Hécaen and Badaraco (1956) do not discuss laterality of lesions; however, their case summaries contain a sufficient number of references to lateralizing signs (in 16 of 24 cases) to permit a comparison: 14 of 16 cases with visual episodes (if these are defined according to our criteria) seem to have a major lesion in the right hemisphere. Further support can be derived from a recent survey from the Montreal Neurological Institute (see Penfield, 1958, p. 220), where it was noted that "visual illusions of alteration (in clearness, distance, nearness, shape, speed of movement, erectness), which occurred during epileptic discharge, arose in the temporal lobe of the nondominant hemisphere, the minor hemisphere for handedness, in 10 out of 11 cases. . . . Stimulation produced these illusions only in the minor hemisphere for handedness. . . ."

Besides a pattern of localization in the lesser hemisphere, visual attacks present a number of qualitative features of considerable interest. Among these are multiple or recurrent vision, distortions in the three-dimensional organization of objects seen, illusory movements, and, in rare cases, formed visual hallucinations.

Episodes of Monocular Diplopia

We have mentioned before (p. 16) that two of our three cases with altitudinal hemianopia (cases A-140 and A-102, though not case A-71, just reviewed) presented monocular double vision, transient in one (A-140) and persistent in the other (A-102); however, in the second case, visual attacks were characterized by an episodic enhancement of this monocular diplopia. We shall briefly describe these attacks for both cases.

The first patient (case A-140), with inferior altitudinal hemianopia resulting from a tangential wound crossing the midline in the midparietal area, still has visual attacks occurring a few times a week; they have remained unchanged in frequency or character since the year of his injury (1944). He describes them as a "flickering, or rather slowly pulsating sensation" in the center of the field of vision, but below the fixation point (i.e., in his blind field), in rainbow colors—"like a slowly turning diamond held against the light." In addition, the episodes are frequently associated with disturbances of form perception in the intact portion of his field: while "flickering" occurs in the lower (blind) half of his field, contours of every object seen in the upper, intact half of the field are temporarily doubled. This diplopia is clearly monocular—the patient reported spontaneously that he saw double contours, regardless of whether he used both eyes, or the left or right eye alone.

In case A-140 the visual episodes were never associated with headaches or dizziness; they evoked no particular distress. However, in case A-102, in which the patient also exhibits an inferior altitudinal defect (see Figs. 6a,b), the episodes are always accompanied by tingling and numbness in both legs and usually by temporary difficulties in speaking and understanding speech. Often there are occipital headaches, dizziness, and nausea. The visual component of the attacks is again nearly identical with that of the previously cited cases. There are flickering phosphenes in the blind region, together with hazy vision and marked diplopia in the less impaired portion. In this case the episodes last from minutes to several hours, and sometimes progress to partial or complete blindness, clearing in several minutes. When attacks of this sort were witnessed by one of us, it was noticed that there was transient bulging of the occipital defect, lasting as long as the attack.

Six years after the patient was wounded, the tantalum plate was removed from the area of defect following a week of increased bulging and tenderness in the occipital region, which were associated with almost hourly recurrence of the diplopia. An epidural granuloma was noted beneath the plate; the dura was not incised. At first the attacks diminished following this operation, but soon were recurring at the rate of several times a month.

Complex Perceptual Changes during Attack

In another of our cases (A-104) transient visual disturbances were also associated with palpable change in the area of the old occipital injury (eventually leading to a transient visible bulging in the area of the defect which was not covered by any plate). However, in contrast to the cases already described, the episodes started in this particular instance seven years after the wounding, became more frequent and more severe over a period of two weeks, and then subsided, without recurrence. Case A-104 is further instructive because it was possible on three separate occasions to obtain electro-encephalographic recordings during a visual episode.

Originally, this patient showed nothing but an insular scotoma in the left parafoveal region (illustrated in Fig. 33), the result of a penetrating wound of the right occipital protuberance. The visual paroxysms began in the eighth year after the wounding, with an episodic distortion of contours: every object in the homonymous left half-field seemed pulled out of shape, obliquely downward and to the lower left. At the same time, those portions of objects that were projected into the affected half-field "looked definitely larger, and the other side smaller than they should look." Attacks of this sort lasted a few seconds, and occurred several times a day.

As the attacks became more frequent and more severe, flicker was noticed by the patient in the area of his scotoma, and objects were perceived "as if in section" or overlaid by a grid. Still later in the course of the disorder (about two weeks from the onset), attacks were occurring with surprising regularity about three times every half-hour and were accompanied not only by multiplication of contours and recurrent vision, but also by sudden disarticulations in visual space, so that entire objects seemed to "bob back and forth."

In this instance, polyopia (multiple vision) was in fact a form of palinopia, that is, of recurrent vision: the patient complained that during attacks moving patterns were seen by him in different places simultaneously, as if he were looking at successive frames of a film (with the film held stationary). For instance, when an examiner rose from a chair to approach him, the patient exclaimed that he perceived the examiner simultaneously as seated and as stepping out towards him. A similar kind of recurrent vision has been described by a patient of Spalding and Zangwill (1950). The phenomena are identical with those reviewed by Critchley (1951) under the designation paliopsia (although we prefer the term palinopia by analogy with such other compound words as palinode, or palindrome).[4]

Electro-encephalographic Changes Correlated with Visual Attacks

In our case A-104 the EEG tracings obtained between the patient's attacks were consistently normal; however, at the beginning of each subjective episode, there appeared a focal discharge consisting of fast activity with gradually increasing amplitude, restricted to the right temporo-occipital region (Figs. 55a,b). About 20 sec. from its onset, the focal activity slowed down without diminishing in amplitude and continued at 3 to 5 per sec. In some instances the abnormal discharge in the EEG disappeared at the time the patient indicated that his subjective visual phenomena had subsided (Fig. 55c); on one occasion, however, the EEG discharge seemed to outlast the subjective episode by a quarter of a minute.

Visual Hallucinations

Despite the high incidence and frequent recurrence of visual aurae of various sorts, frank visual hallucinations were quite rare in our series of cases with field defects resulting from penetrating gunshot wounds. Formed visual hallucinations are perhaps more likely to occur in the presence of posterior lobe abcesses; they have also been observed by us in cases of deep temporo-parietal lesions in which somehow the visual fields had escaped without demonstrable deficits (see also Hécaen and Badaraco, 1956).

An approximation to a hallucinated state was found in only one case of field defect (A-144); this patient, an excellent witness, had been a professional draftsman and cartoonist prior to his induction into the service. He was

---

[4] In another, more recent study from the National Hospital, Queen Square, in London, phenomena quite similar to those seen in our case A-104 were reported (Ettlinger, Warrington, and Zangwill, 1957). With regard to case 9 of their group (that of a scientist with metastatic carcinoma of the right parietal region), the authors say (*loc. cit.,* p. 352): "Prior to radiation therapy, the patient presented for a time more extensive disturbances, marked by formed hallucinations, visual perseveration in the left half-fields, neglect of the left half of extra-personal space, dressing dyspraxia and conceptual spatial loss. Topographical memory was not affected. Two years later, all these symptoms had receded . . . only minimal indications of visual-constructive defect were elicited. . . ." The extent of recovery in this case is nearly as great as in our cases of gunshot wound (group A). Whether "visuo-constructive defects," at these late stages, remain as specific sequelae of occipito-parietal, or even right occipito-parietal lesions (as suggested by Hécaen, Ajuriaguerra, and Massonet, 1951; see also Paterson and Zangwill, 1944), it is difficult to decide for our cases in group A (Teuber and Weinstein, 1954). Nor is it clear whether combined thalamic and cortical lesions play a role in the disarticulations of visual space (as suggested by Herrmann and Pötzl, 1928), or whether activation of central vestibular representations might be involved in these perceptual disturbances (Morsier and Broccard, 1937; Hécaen, Ajuriaguerra, and Massonet, 1951). Critchley has pointed out (1953) that this role of postulated vestibular representations, while possible, is far from proven.

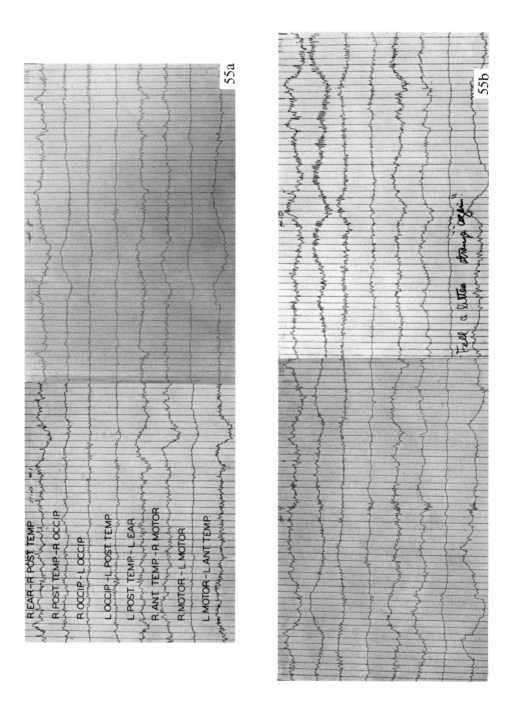

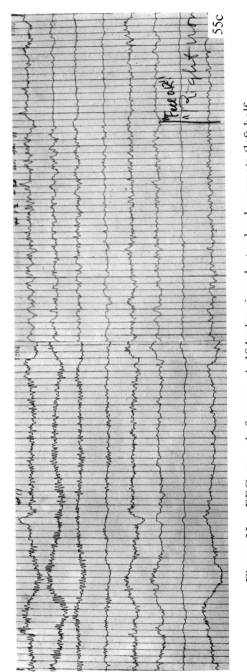

Figure 55a. EEG records for case A-104, showing electrode placements (left half of figure) and essentially normal record in the early part of the recording (right half).

Figure 55b. Gradual onset of focal discharge initially restricted to the right posterior temporal and right occipital regions, consisting of fast activity which increases in amplitude. Notation on record indicates that the patient said, "Feel a little strange again."

Figure 55c. About 20 secs. after the beginning of the focal discharge, the activity in the right temporal and occipital regions slows down without diminishing in amplitude (left half of figure) and continues at 3–5 per sec. (right half). At this point, the patient said, "Feel OK, right now." At the same time, the EEG became essentially normal.

109

wounded by a sniper bullet, which apparently implicated both occipital poles. According to his description, there was an immediate and total blindness, but vision returned during the first two weeks in the usual sequence—first shadows, then contours, then colors, with characteristic confusions between blue and green, and a predominance of red in the early stages of returning color vision. During this time the patient was aware of a marked distortion of shapes; the disturbance was not episodic but more or less continuous throughout the first eight months after the wounding.

His present field defects consist of a total loss of the homonymous left lower quadrant, a partial loss in the left upper quadrant, and some encroachment on the right lower quadrants by an arc which curves from the blind area in the left lower quadrants upwards until it reaches the right horizontal meridian. Because of the persistent dysmorphopsiae, the patient gave up drawing after his discharge from the service, took up writing, and became a fairly successful novelist.

He has given us several written descriptions of his visual attacks. They invariably begin with a slowly pulsating, iridescent light in the blind area of the field. As the pulsation increases in frequency, the intact portion of the left field becomes blind. At the same time there are distortions of contours in the remaining (right) part of the field; these distortions are essentially a transient revival of the dysmorphopsiae which the patient experienced continuously during the first eight months after his injury.

It is at this stage during some attacks that the patient has what he himself regards as hallucinations. He writes, "I rarely see things in the blind area but I become aware of them—I keep trying to see them, till I get nauseated." In these situations, the patient apparently experiences the *presque vu* phenomenon which has previously been described (e.g., Klüver, 1928, 1942b). He feels that he is about to see something but fails to perceive it. He continues: "The only things I can remember ever getting near enough to presume to name were a tall, wide barn door that changed to a wire gate of similar dimensions, and a very colorful fowl."

Such formed visual hallucinations can be a considerable hazard to the patient, even if he remains convinced of their lack of reality. One of our patients, who was injured by the passage of a bullet from the left temporal through the right parietal region but who had no field defect, was seized with grand mal convulsions several times a year. The attack always began with a visual hallucination, clearly polyopic in character. The patient would see a train of small horses, in many colors, similar to a series of wooden horses on a merry-go-round. These appeared in the periphery of his field, on the left, and moved towards the center, where they disappeared. This visual symptom was followed in most instances by a grand mal seizure, after which the patient exhibited some postictal confusion and moderate aphasia, which cleared within a few minutes to several hours. Following one of these attacks, he was picked up by the police under suspicion of either drunkenness or drug addiction; after a few hours, during which the patient tried to explain his condition in a somewhat dysphasic fashion, it was decided to send him to a State hospital. There the patient was kept under observation; eventually, he confided in a staff member (upon insistent questioning with regard to visual hallucinations) that he occasionally saw "horses." The result was a two-year period of hospitalization, entirely unnecessary in this case, under the diagnosis of "schizophrenia with visual hallucinations and occasional word salad."

Implications of Visual Fits

We have described in detail some of the visual aurae experienced by patients in group A because in many ways they represent a recurrence of the continuous visual distortions noted in patients of group SD, whom we observed shortly after they had sustained penetrating missile wounds of the posterior brain substance. In our earlier reports based on group SD (e.g., Bender and Teuber, 1947b, 1948), we had described various forms of persistent distortion of visual space experienced by these patients. The distortions consisted predominantly of an increase in the apparent distance of objects seen (teleopsia), often associated with a decrease in their apparent size (micropsia). In some cases, movement in the visual field or movement of the eye produced multiple vision (monocular diplopia or polyopia; see Bender, 1945). All these disturbances were limited to homonymous areas of the visual field: they appeared in half-fields, quadrants, or sectors of quadrants. Some day-to-day fluctuation in severity of symptoms was noted, but all patients exhibited the disorder continuously throughout the period of observation, which lasted up to one year following trauma.

It was our impression, at that time, that many cases of gunshot wounds implicating the geniculocalcarine sector showed these disturbances in the early stages after injury (see also Mingazzini, 1908; Chatelin and Patrikios, 1917). Yet we did not know whether the symptoms, once present, tended to persist continuously and indefinitely. The observations made in group A seem to indicate that the disorder gradually disappears, but is likely to recur during certain episodes, or "visual attacks." These conclusions would be consistent with earlier comments made from various sides (e.g., Hebb, 1950) to the effect that the continuous distortions in visual space observed in group SD might have reflected the persistence of irritative phenomena in the brain, rather than the mere absence of cerebral tissue. However, these disordered perceptions remain instructive, regardless of whether one attributes them to irritative phenomena or not. It is further noteworthy that these persistent early distortions as well as their episodic recurrence should be so similar to the visual changes reported in migraine attacks (Beyer, 1895; Rønne, 1936; Weeks, 1940; Lashley, 1941; Rich, 1948) or toxic states, especially mescal intoxication (Beringer, 1927; Klüver, 1928, 1942b; Zádor, 1930).

The problem of relationships between attacks of migraine and epileptic manifestations is as old as it is unresolved. Gowers (1907) proposed that visual disturbances in migraine differed basically from those seen in visual fits. Although both types of episodes may be characterized by a "march" (i.e., a definite sequence of disturbances in each episode), Gowers thought that the march was much quicker in epileptic than in migraine attacks. This distinction may apply in some but certainly not in all of our cases of visual fits. In case A-144, for instance, the "march" was as slow and prolonged as in many cases of "ordinary migraine."

These similarities suggest that the visual system responds with a rather uniform pattern to seemingly dissimilar abnormal states. Continued study of such stereotyped disorders of perception may bring us closer to an understanding of normal visual physiology.

8. Summary and Conclusions

Visual fields were studied by a standardized perimetric method in 203 cases of missile wounds of the brain; with few exceptions, the injuries had been sustained from 5 to 10 years prior to testing. Visual fields were found to be defective in 46 cases of the 203; these 46 were subjected to additional field examinations by perimetry, campimetry, and various adjunct methods, including flicker perimetry. Since visual field examinations were done repeatedly in every case, the results permitted an estimate of the repeat-reliability of the perimetric method, which was found to be high. At the same time, the results showed a remarkable persistence of these field defects due to gunshot wounds; if one excludes episodes of visual attacks with transient changes in the visual field, the defects found were unchanged for decades. Twenty-four of the 46 defective fields are illustrated. For purposes of comparison and contrast, 9 additional cases from earlier studies involving acute after-effects of wounds of the visual pathways have been discussed, and 8 of these are illustrated.

The results were analyzed with regard to the classic principle of retino-topical projection. We asked to what extent the shape and nature of the field defects observed could have been predicted on the basis of existing concepts of visual anatomy. While some results could have been predicted in this way, others could not.

Among the results confirmatory of earlier studies were the following:

Tangential wounds crossing the midline slightly above the occipital poles tended to produce inferior altitudinal hemianopiae, either complete or incomplete. Superior altitudinal hemianopiae, however, were absent in our group, just as they have been found rarely, if ever, in earlier studies of penetrating trauma.

Destruction in the presumed region of both occipital poles can lead to selective loss of the entire macular region; conversely, penetrating wounds through the posterior lobe substance directed somewhat more anteriorly may be followed by permanent bilateral hemianopia with macular sparing (peephole vision).

There were a number of instances of concentric contraction of the visual field; in these cases the boundary between blind and less-impaired portions of the field was fairly irregular. This irregular outline was maintained, and the diameter of the less-impaired portion of the field increased, when the field was plotted at one distance on a tangent screen, and the patient then moved farther away, and the field replotted. This finding contrasted with an illustrative case of hysterical tunnel vision; here the field taken at twice the original distance was smaller in diameter (rather than larger), and exhibited smooth circular outlines on both occasions.

There was a high incidence (7 in 46) of small insular defects, often wedge-shaped and pointing towards the fovea. Such wedge-shaped defects were found with penetration impinging on the occiput, but were also present in cases in which the wound of entrance and the path of the missile suggested that the injury was in the optic radiation.

In a number of instances, the monocular crescent was selectively spared or selectively lost; this was also true for "quadrantic" portions of the crescent. Quadrantic defects filling exactly one quadrant of the visual field were not found in this series. The defects either amounted to less than a quadrant and then were sector-shaped (tapering towards the fovea) or extended beyond the confines of a single quadrant. However, no consistent pattern of sparing of horizontal meridians (as described by Spalding) could be demonstrated.

In agreement with Spalding (and contrary to Polyak) we believe that the varied shapes of field defects after penetrating wounds of the optic radiation may require a revision of current views regarding the intrinsic organization of this part of the central visual pathways. Evidence is presented which suggests that the macular fibers cannot form a distinct bundle coursing at intermediate height between ventral and dorsal bundles representing, respectively, the upper and lower peripheral quadrants of the visual field. At least in the anterior parts of man's optic radiation, the macular fibers seem to overlap with these peripheral representations.

In hemianopic defects some amount of macular sparing was observed for 15 cases, and complete macular splitting in the remaining 3. Data are presented to show that the varied instances of sparing do not have a common origin.

The appearance of sparing is attributed to any or all of three factors: (1) eccentric fixation, including persistent use of a pseudo-fovea (as an objective indication of the existence of pseudo-fovea, we employed the abnormal position of the blind spot); (2) lack of congruence between homonymous monocular fields (see below); (3) lower vulnerability of the central fields as against the peripheral fields, owing to widespread macular representation in optic radiation and cortex and, possibly, to better vascular supply of the cortical macula.

The principal finding at variance with a majority of previous reports is the lack of congruence of homonymous field defects. We could not confirm Henschen's notion of an "almost mathematical congruence" of homonymous field defects (the more so, he thought, the closer the lesion approached the striate cortex).

One factor in the production of incongruent field defects was the tendency for defects in a nasal field to appear larger or denser on perimetry than the corresponding (homonymous) defect in the temporal field of the other eye. Paradoxically, the patient usually experienced the lesser defect (in the temporal half) as the more serious one, or as the one that disturbed him most. In addition, we found a general lack of congruence (as to detail) in the outlines of homonymous field defects. This was true regardless of the localization of the wounds of entrance which produced the defects. The most probable interpretation of this incongruence would be that, contrary to current anatomic conceptions, corresponding elements in the visual system are not perfectly aligned, even at the level of the striate cortex.

The report has likewise stressed that in hemianopic defects the division between the blind and the seeing field rarely forms a straight line. Here, too, irregularities in the course of the dividing line appear, and these are different when the two monocular fields are compared.

In the series of cases studied, nearly all of the scotomata were negative, that is, they were not experienced as an area of darkness, or a positive void. Some of the claw-shaped parafoveal defects are exceptions to this statement, since they were experienced by the patient as faint lines interposed between them and the objects they fixated. Although the scotomata as such were negative, the patient did not in any instance deny their existence after the fashion of denial of blindness in diffuse cerebral disease. Even when the injury produced an initial total blindness, as often happened (7 out of 46 cases), the patient reacted appropriately.

In everyday activities, the patients' awareness of their scotomata was further diminished by the occurrence of completion effects. The report summarizes results of experiments showing the completion of apparent movement across blind areas, and it discusses other ways in which completion of contours makes the patients' functioning fields seemingly wider than the perimetric fields. By contrast, extinction effects diminish the functioning field wherever vision in an impaired region is momentarily lost on intercurrent stimulation of some other, less-impaired region.

Despite the widespread occurrence of completion effects, some of these scotomata can become entoptically visible. Several of the patients with claw-shaped defects reported that on fixating a red background, their scotomata appeared to them in green. When an after-image of the red background had developed and was projected on a neutral gray screen, the scotoma itself appeared in red, while the surround, that is the after-image of the background, appeared in green.

The shape of color fields was generally found to duplicate the outline of fields for form and motion but with a much shorter diameter. These and similar results seem to us to indicate that while different areas of the visual field are projected to approximately corresponding loci in the higher visual pathway, the various levels of visual function are not so represented.

In line with this interpretation are results obtained by means of auxiliary methods of assessing visual fields, for example, flicker perimetry. In the presence of circumscribed field defects, there were subtle but significant changes in other visual functions, even in those parts of the field which seemed intact according to the perimetric plot. The seemingly intact half of hemi-anopic fields showed a significant reduction in the fusion thresholds for flickering light; dark adaptation was likewise impaired.

The various circumscribed scotomata thus are essentially compatible with the principle of point-for-point projection of retina into cortex, although details of this projection remain to be worked out. However, as soon as the functioning visual field is considered, this principle of retinotopical projection, as such, needs to be modified: various aspects of visual performance are affected in the presence of circumscribed lesions; their alteration extends over the entire field, and to either side of the midline. These remote effects of seemingly focal lesions may mean either that the lesions are more diffuse than the circumscribed scotomata indicate or that the functions in all parts of the field depend on the integrity of every individual part. We cannot decide between these two views, diffuseness of lesions, or diffuse representation.

The scotoma, as a negative symptom (or sign of loss of function), points at specificity of representation; if we have stressed gaps and inconsistencies in current anatomic knowledge of orderly projection, we have done so because this knowledge can be made more specific and more complete. Yet no matter how precise our grasp of the structure, an understanding of visual physiology needs to account for the many instances of diffuse interaction within the injured substrate. Among these positive effects of the lesions are the visuospatial disorders during acute stages after occipital injury; the recurrence of these disorders, in the form of visual fits, in later years; the persistence of subtle but systematic alterations in visual function in all cases of scotoma, and in every part of their field. While these observations do not, by themselves, suggest a theory, any theory of vision will have to take them into account.

References

ADLER, ALEXANDRA (1941). Disintegration and restoration of optic recognition in visual agnosia, *Arch. Neurol. Psychiat. (Chicago)* 45:788–796.

ADLER, ALEXANDRA (1950). Course and outcome of visual agnosia, *J. nerv. ment. Dis.* 111:41–51.

ALLEN, I. M. (1930). A clinical study of tumours involving the occipital lobe, *Brain* 53:194–243.

ANTON, G. (1898). Ueber Herderkrankungen des Gehirns, welche vom Patienten selbst nicht wahrgenommen werden, *Wien. klin. Wschr.* 11:227–229.

AUSTIN, G. M., LEWEY, F. H., and GRANT, F. C. (1949). Studies on the occipital lobe: I. Significance of small areas of preserved central vision, *Arch. Neurol. Psychiat. (Chicago)* 62:204–221.

BALADO, M., ADROGUE, E., and FRANKE, ELIZABETH (1928). Contribución al estudio anatómico de las hemianopias en cuadrante, *Bol. Inst. Clín. quirúrg. (B. Aires)* 4 (2):520–535.

BALADO, M., and MALBRAN, J. (1932). Sobre la localización de la mácula en el hombre, *Arch. Oftal. B. Aires* 7:259–278.

BALADO, M., MALBRAN, J., and FRANKE, ELIZABETH (1934). Doble incongruencia hemianópsica de origen cortical (estudio anatómo-clínico), *Arch. argent. Neurol.* 10:201–212.

BALINT, R. (1909). Seelenlähmung des Schauens, *Mschr. Psychiat. Neurol.* 25:51–81.

BÁRÁNY, R. (1924). La bipartition de la couche interne des grains, est-elle l'expression anatomique de la réprésentation isolée des champs visuels monoculaires dans l'écorce cérébrale? *Trab. Lab. Invest. biol. Univ. Madr.* 22:359–368.

BATTERSBY, W. S. (1951). The regional gradient of critical flicker frequency after frontal or occipital injury, *J. exp. Psychol.* 42:59–68.

BATTERSBY, W. S., BENDER, M. B., and TEUBER, H.-L. (1951). Effects of total light flux on critical flicker frequency after frontal lobe lesion, *J. exp. Psychol.* 42:135–142.

BATTERSBY, W. S., and BENDER, M. B. (1958). Temporal determinants of foveal CFF after lesions of the cerebral visual pathways, *J. comp. physiol. Psychol.* 51:411–416.

BATTERSBY, W. S., and WAGMAN, I. H. (1959). Alterations of visual excitability in patients with lesions of the central optic pathways, *Trans. Amer. neurol. Ass.*, 84th ann. mtg., pp. 156–159.

BAY, E. (1950). *Agnosie und Funktionswandel; eine hirnpathologische Studie.* Berlin: Springer.

BAY, E. (1953). Disturbances of visual perception and their examination, *Brain* 76:515–550.

BAY, E. (1954). Optische Faktoren bei den räumlichen Orientierungsstörungen, *Dtsch. Z. Nervenheilk.* 171:454–459.

BEHR, C. (1931). Die Erkrankungen der Sehbahn vom Chiasma aufwärts. In *Kurzes Handbuch der Ophthalmologie* (ed. F. Schieck and A. Brückner), vol. VI: *Auge und Nervensystem*, pp. 245–323. Berlin: Springer.

BENDER, M. B. (1945). Polyopia and monocular diplopia of cerebral origin, *Arch. Neurol. Psychiat. (Chicago)* 54:323–338.

BENDER, M. B. (1952). *Disorders in Perception.* Springfield, Ill.: Thomas.

BENDER, M. B., and BATTERSBY, W. S. (1958). Homonymous macular scotomata in cases of occipital lobe tumor, *Arch. Ophthal. (Chicago)* 60:928–938.

BENDER, M. B., and FURLOW, L. T. (1945a). Phenomenon of visual extinction in homonymous fields and psychologic principles involved, *Arch. Neurol. Psychiat. (Chicago)* 53:29–33.

BENDER, M. B., and FURLOW, L. T., (1945b). Visual disturbances produced by bilateral lesions of the occipital lobes with central scotomas, *Arch. Neurol. Psychiat. (Chicago)* 53:165–170.

BENDER, M. B., FURLOW, L. T., and TEUBER, H.-L. (1949). Alterations in behavior after massive cerebral trauma (intraventricular foreign body), *Confin. neurol. (Basel)* 9: 140–157.

BENDER, M. B., and KAHN, R. L. (1949). After-imagery in defective fields of vision, *J. Neurol. Neurosurg. Psychiat* 12:196–204.

BENDER, M. B., and KANZER, M. (1939). Dynamics of homonymous hemianopias and preservation of central vision, *Brain* 62:404–421.

BENDER, M. B., and TEUBER, H.-L. (1946). Phenomena of fluctuation, extinction, and completion in visual perception, *Arch. Neurol. Psychiat. (Chicago)* 55:627–658.

BENDER, M. B., and TEUBER, H.-L. (1947a). Ring scotoma and tubular fields;

their significance in cases of head injury, *Arch. Neurol. Psychiat. (Chicago)* 56:200–226.

BENDER, M. B., and TEUBER, H.-L., (1947b). Spatial organization of visual perception following injury to the brain, *Arch. Neurol. Psychiat. (Chicago)* 58:721–739.

BENDER, M. B., and TEUBER, H.-L. (1948). Spatial organization of visual perception following injury to the brain, *Arch. Neurol. Psychiat. (Chicago)* 59:39–62.

BENDER, M. B., and TEUBER, H.-L. (1949). Psychopathology of vision. Chap. 8 in *Progress in Neurology and Psychiatry,* vol. IV (ed. E. A. Spiegel). New York: Grune & Stratton.

BERINGER, K. (1927). *Der Meskalinrausch, seine Geschichte und Erscheinungsweise* (Monogr. Neurol. Psychiat., no. 49). Berlin: Springer.

BEST, F. (1917). Hemianopsie und Seelenblindheit bei Hirnverletzungen, *Albrecht v. Graefes Arch. Ophthal.* 93:49–150.

BEST, F. (1919). Zur Theorie der Hemianopsie und der höheren Sehzentren, *Albrecht v. Graefes Arch. Ophthal.* 100:1–31.

BEST, F. (1920). Ergebnisse der Kriegsjahre für die Kenntnis der Sehbahnen und Sehzentren, *Zbl. ges. Ophthal.* 3:193–207, 241–254.

BEYER, E. (1895). Ueber Verlagerungen im Gesichtsfeld bei Flimmerskotom, *Neurol. Centralbl. (Lpz.)* 14:10–15.

BIELSCHOWSKY, A. (1931). Der Sehakt bei Störungen im Bewegungsapparat der Augen, *Handb. norm. pathol. Physiol.* (ed. A. Bethe *et al.*), 12 (2):1095–1112. Berlin: Springer.

BLUM, JOSEPHINE (SEMMES), CHOW, K. L., and PRIBRAM, K. H. (1950). A behavioral analysis of the organization of the parieto-temporo-preoccipital cortex, *J. comp. Neurol.* 93:53–100.

BROUWER, B. (1917). Ueber die Sehstrahlung des Menschen, *Mschr. Psychiat. Neurol.* 41:129–158, 203–234.

BROUWER, B. (1930). Ueber die Projektion der Makula auf die Area striata des Menschen, *J. Psychol. Neurol. (Lpz.)* 40:147–159.

BRÜCKNER, A. (1917). Zur Frage der Lokalisation des Kontrastes und verwandter Erscheinungen in der Sehsinnsubstanz, *Z. Augenheilk.* 38:1–14.

BRUNS, L. (1886). Ein Beitrag zur einseitigen Wahrnehmung doppelseitiger Reize bei Herden einer Grosshirnhemisphäre, *Neurol. Centralbl. (Lpz.)* 5:198–199.

CHACKO, L. W. (1948). An analysis of fibre-size in the human optic nerve, *Brit. J. Ophthal.* 32:457–461.

CHARCOT, J. M. (1883). Un cas de suppression brusque et isolé de la vision mentale des signes et des objets (formes et couleurs), *Progr. méd. (Paris)* 11:568–571.

CHATELIN, C., and PATRIKIOS (1917). Phénomènes d'irritation de la sphère visuelle et mal comitial consécutifs à une blessure de la pointe du lobe occipital gauche, *Rev. neurol.* 24:259–261.

CHOW, K. L. (1952a). Further studies on selective ablations of associative cortex in relation to visually mediated behavior, *J. comp. physiol. Psychol.* 45:109–118.

CHOW, K. L. (1952b). Conditions influencing the recovery of visual discriminative habits in monkeys following temporal neocortical ablations, *J. comp. physiol. Psychol.* 45:430–437.

CHOW, K. L., BLUM, JOSEPHINE (SEMMES), and BLUM, R. A. (1950). Cell ratios in the thalamo-cortical visual system of Macaca mulatta, *J. comp. Neurol.* 92:227–240.

CHRISTIAN, P., and SCHMITZ, W. (1942). Untersuchungen von Sehhirnverletzten mit optischen Periodenreizen, *Dtsch. Z. Nervenheilk.* 154:81–131.

CHRISTIAN, P., and UMBACH, W. (1947). Sehschärfe, Beleuchtungshelligkeit, und Riccòscher Satz bei Sehhirnverletzten, *Dtsch. Z. Nervenheilk.* 158:1–15.

CIBIS, P. (1947). Zur Pathologie der Lokaladaptation: I. Physiologische und klinische Untersuchungen zur quantitativen Analyse der örtlichen Umstimmungserscheinungen des Licht- und Farbensinnes unter besonderer Berücksichtigung hirnpathologischer Fälle, *Albrecht v. Graefes Arch. Ophthal.* 148:1–15.

CIBIS, P. (1948). Zur Pathologie der Lokaladaptation: II. Konstruktive Darstellung der Erregungsvorgänge bei konstanter und phasischer Reizung umschriebener Sehfeldstellen, *Albrecht v. Graefes Arch. Ophthal.* 148:216–257.

CIBIS, P., and MÜLLER, H. (1948). Lokaladaptometrische Untersuchungen am Projektionsperimeter nach Maggiore, *Albrecht v. Graefes Arch. Ophthal.* 148:468–489.

CLARK, G. (1948). The mode of representation in the motor cortex, *Brain* 71:332–342.

CLARK, W. E. LE GROS (1941). Observations on the association fiber system of the visual cortex and the central representation of the retina, *J. Anat. (Lond.)* 74:225–235.

COHEN, L. (1959). Perception of reversible figures by normal and brain-injured subjects, *Arch. Neurol. Psychiat. (Chicago)* 81:765–775.

CRITCHLEY, M. (1951). Types of visual perseveration; "paliopsia" and "illusory visual spread," *Brain* 74:267–299.

CRITCHLEY, M. (1953). *The Parietal Lobes.* Baltimore: Williams & Wilkins.

CUSHING, H. (1922). The field defects produced by temporal lobe lesions, *Brain* 44:341–396.

DÉJÉRINE, J., and ROUSSY, G. (1906). Le syndrome thalamique, *Rev. neurol.* 14:521–532.

DENNY-BROWN, D. (1951). The frontal lobes and their functions. Chap. 2 in *Modern Trends in Neurology* (ed. A. Feiling). New York: Hoeber.

DENNY-BROWN, D., and BOTTERELL, E. H. (1948). The motor functions of the agranular frontal cortex, *Res. Publ. Ass. nerv. ment. Dis.* 27:235–245.

DOTY, R. W. (1958). Potentials evoked in cat cerebral cortex by diffuse and by punctiform photic stimuli, *J. Neurophysiol.* 21:437–464.

DUKE-ELDER, SIR W. S. (1949). *Text-book of Ophthalmology,* vol. IV: *The Neurology of Vision; Motor and Optical Anomalies.* London: Kimpton.

ETTLINGER, G. (1959). Visual discrimination following successive temporal ablations in monkeys, *Brain* 82:232–250.

ETTLINGER, G., WARRINGTON, ELIZABETH, and ZANGWILL, O. L. (1957). A further study of visual-spatial agnosia, *Brain* 80:335–361.

EVARTS, E. V. (1952). Effects of ablation of prestriate cortex on auditory-visual association in monkeys, *J. Neurophysiol.* 15:191–200

FALCONER, M. A., and WILSON, J. L. (1958). Visual field changes following anterior temporal lobectomy; their significance in relation to "Meyer's loop" of the optic radiation, *Brain* 81:1–14.

FAUST, C. (1947a). Ueber Gestaltzerfall als Symptom des parieto-occipitalen Uebergangsgebietes bei doppelseitiger Verletzung nach Hirnschuss, *Nervenarzt* 18:103–115.

FAUST, C. (1947b). Partielle Seelenblindheit nach Occipitalhirnverletzung mit besonderer Beeinträchtigung des Physiognomieerkennens, *Nervenarzt* 18:294–297.

FAUST, C. (1955). *Die zerebralen Herdstörungen bei Hinterhauptsverletzungen und ihre Beurteilung* (Arbeit und Gesundheit, n.s., no. 57). Stuttgart: Thieme.

FEINBERG, I. (1956). Critical flicker frequency in amblyopia ex anopsia, *Amer. J. Ophthal.* 42:473–481.

FERREE, C. E., and RAND, G. (1919). Chromatic thresholds of sensation from center to periphery of the retina and their bearing on color theory, *Psychol. Rev.* 26:16–41.

FLEISCHER, B. (1916). Ueber den Ausfall bzw. die Erhaltung des nur von einem Auge bestrittenen sichelförmigen Aussenteils des binokularen Gesichtsfeldes (des "temporalen Halbmondes") durch Schussverletzung (abstract), *Klin. Mbl. Augenheilk.* 57:140.

FOERSTER, O. (1929). Beiträge zur Pathophysiologie der Sehbahn und der Sehsphäre, *J. Psychol. Neurol. (Lpz.)* 39:463–485.

FÖRSTER, R. (1867). Ueber Gesichtsfeldmessungen, *Klin. Mbl. Augenheilk.* 5:293–294.

FÖRSTER, R. (1890). Ueber Rindenblindheit, *Albrecht v. Graefes Arch. Ophthal.* 36:94–108.

FOX, J. C., JR., and GERMAN, W. J. (1936). Macular vision following cerebral resection, *Arch. Neurol. Psychiat. (Chicago)* 35:808–826.

FRANZ, S. I. (1923). *Nervous and Mental Reeducation.* New York: Macmillan.

FRANZ, S. I., and ODEN, R. (1917). On cerebral motor control; the recovery from experimentally produced hemiplegia, *Psychobiol.* 1:3–18.

FREUD, S. (1891). *Zur Auffassung der Aphasien; eine kritische Studie.* Leipzig: Deuticke.

FUCHS, W. (1920). Untersuchungen über das Sehen der Hemianopiker und Hemiamblyopiker: I. Verlagerungserscheinungen, *Z. Psychol.* 84:67–169.

FUCHS, W. (1921). Untersuchungen über das Sehen der Hemianopiker und Hemiamblyopiker: II. Die totalisierende Gestaltauffassung, *Z. Psychol.* 86:1–143.

FUCHS, W. (1922). Eine Pseudofovea bei Hemianopikern, *Psychol. Forsch.* 1:157–186.

FURLOW, L. T., BENDER, M. B., and TEUBER, H.-L. (1947). Movable foreign body within the cerebral ventricle, *J. Neurosurg.* 4:380–386.

GELB, A., and GOLDSTEIN, K. (1920 sqq.). *Psychologische Analysen hirnpathologischer Fälle.* Leipzig: Barth. (Parts translated in W. D. Ellis, *A Source Book of Gestalt Psychology.* New York: Harcourt, 1938.)

GELB, A., and GOLDSTEIN, K. (1922). Psychologische Analysen hirnpathologischer Fälle auf Grund von Untersuchungen Hirnverletzter: VII. Ueber Gesichtsfeldbefunde bei abnormer "Ermüdbarkeit" des Auges (sog. "Ringskotome"), *Albrecht v. Graefes Arch. Ophthal.* 109:387–403.

GHENT, LILA, WEINSTEIN, S., SEMMES, JOSEPHINE, and TEUBER, H.-L. (1955). Effect of unilateral brain injury in man on learning of a tactual discrimination, *J. comp. physiol. Psychol.* 48:478–481.

GIBSON, J. J. (1950). *The Perception of the Visual World.* Boston: Houghton Mifflin.

GLEES, P., and NAUTA, W. J. H. (1955). A critical review of studies on axonal and terminal degeneration, *Mschr. Psychiat. Neurol.* 129:74–91.

GOLDSTEIN, K. (1927). Die Lokalisation in der Grosshirnrinde. In *Handb. norm. pathol. Physiol.* (ed. A. Bethe *et al.*), 10:600–842. Berlin: Springer.

GOLDSTEIN, K. (1934). Ueber monokuläre Doppelbilder, *Jb. Psychiat. Neurol.* 51:16–38.

GOLDSTEIN, K. (1942). *After-Effects of Brain Injuries in War.* New York: Grune & Stratton.

GOLDSTEIN, K. (1943). Constriction of visual fields, *Arch. Neurol. Psychiat. (Chicago)* 50:486–487.

GOLDSTEIN, K., and GELB, A. (1918). Das "röhrenförmige Gesichtsfeld" nebst einer Vorrichtung für perimetrische Gesichtsfelduntersuchungen in verschiedenen Entfernungen, *Neurol. Centralbl. (Lpz.)* 37:738–748.

GOTTSCHALDT, K. (1926). Ueber den Einfluss der Erfahrung auf die Wahrnehmung von Figuren, *Psychol. Forsch.* 8:261–317.

GOTTSCHALDT, K. (1929). Ueber den Einfluss der Erfahrung auf die Wahrnehmung von Figuren, *Psychol. Forsch.* 12:1–87.

GOWERS, W. R. C. (1907). *Borderland of Epilepsy.* Philadelphia: Blakiston.

HALSTEAD, W. C. (1947). *Brain and Intelligence; a Quantitative Study of the Frontal Lobes.* Chicago: Univ. of Chicago Press.

HALSTEAD, W. C., WALKER, A. E., and BUCY, P. C. (1940). Sparing and nonsparing of "macular" vision associated with occipital lobectomy in man, *Arch. Ophthal. (Chicago)* 24:948–962.

HARLOW, H. F. (1939). Recovery of pattern discrimination in monkeys following unilateral occipital lobectomy, *J. comp. Physiol.* 27:467–489.

HARMAN, P. J., and TEUBER, H.-L. (1959). The geniculo-calcarine system of M. R.; a case of cortical blindness. Paper read at Spring meeting of American Anatomists, Seattle, Washington.

HARRINGTON, D. O. (1939). Localizing value of incongruity in defects in the visual fields, *Arch. Ophthal. (New York)* 21:453–464.

HEAD, H. (1920). *Studies in Neurology.* London: Oxford Medical Publications.

HEBB, D. O. (1950). Animal and physiological psychology, *Ann. Rev. Psychol.* 1:173–188.

HEBEL, K., and LUTHER, EVA (1947). Ueber Nachbilduntersuchungen an Hirnverletzten unter Zugrundelegung normalphysiologischer Experimente, *Dtsch. Z. Nervenheilk.* 158:16–42.

HÉCAEN, H., AJURIAGUERRA, J. DE, and MASSONET, J. (1951). Les troubles visuoconstructifs par lésion pariéto-occipitale droite; rôle des perturbations vestibulaires, *Encéphale* 40:122–179.

HÉCAEN, H., and BADARACO, J. G. (1956). Séméiologie des hallucinations visuelles en clinique neurologique, *Acta neurol. lat.-amer.* 2:23–57.

HECHT, S., and SHLAER, S. (1938). Adaptometer for measuring human dark adaptation, *J. opt. Soc. Amer.* 28:269–275.

HEINE, L. (1900). Sehschärfe und Tiefenwahrnehmung, *Albrecht v. Graefes Arch. Ophthal.* 51:146–173.

HENSCHEN, S. E. (1910). Die zentralen Sehstörungen. In *Handbuch der Neurologie* (ed. M. Lewandowsky), 1:891–918. Berlin: Springer.

HENSCHEN, S. E. (1911). *Klinische und anatomische Beiträge zur Pathologie des Gehirns*, part IV. Uppsala: Almquist Wiksell.

HENSCHEN, S. E. (1923). Vierzigjähriger Kampf um das Sehzentrum und seine Bedeutung für die Hirnforschung, *Z. ges. Neurol. Psychiat.* 87:505–535.

HERRMANN, G., and PÖTZL, O. (1928). *Die optische Allaesthesie.* Berlin: Karger.

HINES, MARION. (1942). Recent contributions to localization of vision in the central nervous system, *Arch. Ophthal. (Chicago)* 28:913–937.

HOLMES, G. (1918a). Disturbances of vision by cerebral lesions, *Brit. J. Ophthal.* 2:353–384.

HOLMES, G. (1918b). Disturbances of visual orientation, *Brit. J. Ophthal.* 2:449–468, 506–516.

HOLMES, G. (1919a). The cortical localization of vision, *Brit. med. J.* 2:193–199.

HOLMES, G. (1919b). Disturbances of visual space perception, *Brit. med. J.* 2:230–233.

HOLMES, G. (1931). A contribution to the cortical representation of vision, *Brain* 54:470–479.

HOLMES, G. (1934). The representation of the mesial sectors of the retinae in the calcarine cortex, *Jb. Psychiat. Neurol.* 51:39–48.

HOLMES, G. (1945). The organization of the visual cortex in man (Ferrier Lecture, delivered May 18, 1944), *Proc. roy. Soc. B* 132:348–361.

HOLMES, G., and LISTER, W. T. (1916). Disturbances of vision from cerebral lesions, with special reference to the cortical representation of the macula, *Brain* 39:34–73.

HORRAX, G., and PUTNAM, T. J. (1932). Distortions of the visual fields in cases of brain tumor: VII. The field defects and hallucinations produced by tumors of the occipital lobe, *Brain* 55:499–523.

HUBEL, D. H. (1959). Cortical unit responses to visual stimuli in unanesthetized cats, *Amer. J. Ophthal.* 46:110–122.

HUGHES, E. B. C. (1954). *The Visual Fields; a Study of the Applications of Quantitative Perimetry to the Anatomy and Pathology of the Visual Pathways.* Springfield, Ill.: Thomas.

HYNDMAN, O. R. (1939). The central visual system; evidence against bilateral representation through splenium of the corpus callosum, *Arch. Neurol. Psychiat. (Chicago)* 42:735–742.

IGERSHEIMER, J. (1919). Zur Pathologie der Sehbahn: IV. Gesichtsfeldverbesserung bei Hemianopikern, *Albrecht v. Graefes Arch. Ophthal.* 100:357–369.

INOUYE, T. (1909). *Die Sehstörungen nach Schussverletzungen der kortikalen Sehsphäre, nach Beobachtungen an Verwundeten der letzten japanischen Kriege.* Leipzig: Engelmann.

IRIS, F. M. (1956). *Contribution à l'étude du rétrécissement concentrique du champ visuel dans le syndrome commotionel des traumatisés du crâne* (Thèse de Paris). Paris: Taib.

JUNG, R. (1948). Symposion über die Grundlagen der Hirnpathologie, *Nervenarzt* 19:518–529.

JUNG, R. (1958). Coordination of specific and nonspecific afferent impulses at single neurons of the visual cortex. Chap. 21 in *The Reticular Formation of the Brain* (ed. H. H. Jasper et al.). Boston: Little, Brown.

KEEN, W. W., and THOMSON, W. (1871). Gunshot-wound of the brain, followed by fungus cerebri, and recovery with hemiopsia, *Trans. Amer. ophthal. Soc.,* 8th mtg., pp. 122–127.

KLEIST, K. (1926). Die einzeläugigen Gesichtsfelder und ihre Vertretung in den beiden Lagern der verdoppelten inneren Körnerschicht der Sehrinde, *Klin. Wschr.* 5:3–10.

KLEIST, K. (1934). *Gehirnpathologie.* Leipzig: Barth.

KLÜVER, H. (1927). Visual disturbances after cerebral lesions, *Psychol. Bull.* 24:316–358.

KLÜVER, H. (1928). *Mescal; the "Divine" Plant and Its Psychological Effects.* London: Paul, Trench, Trubner.

KLÜVER, H. (1937). Certain effects of lesions of the occipital lobes in macaques, *J. of Psychol.* 4:383–401.

KLÜVER, H. (1941). Visual functions after removal of the occipital lobes, *J. of Psychol.* 11:23–45.

KLÜVER, H. (1942a). Functional significance of the geniculo-striate system. In *Biol. Sympos.* (ed. H. Klüver), 7:253–299.

KLÜVER, H. (1942b). Mechanisms of hallucinations. Chap. X in *Studies in Personality.* New York: McGraw-Hill.

KLÜVER, H., and BUCY, P. C. (1938). An analysis of certain effects of bilateral temporal lobectomy in the rhesus monkey, with special reference to "psychic blindness," *J. of Psychol.* 5:33–54.

KLÜVER, H., and BUCY, P. C. (1939). Preliminary analysis of functions of the temporal lobes in monkeys, *Arch. Neurol. Psychiat. (Chicago)* 42:979–1000.

KOFFKA, K. (1935). *Principles of Gestalt Psychology.* New York: Harcourt.

KOHLER, I. (1951). Ueber Aufbau und Wandlung der Wahrnehmungswelt; insbesondere über "bedingte Empfindungen," *S.B. öst. Akad. Wiss., Phil.-hist. Kl.,* vol. 227, no. 1. Vienna: Rohrer.

KÖHLER, W. (1940). *Dynamics in Psychology.* New York: Liveright.

KÖHLER, W., and HELD, R. (1949). The cortical correlate of pattern vision, *Science* 110:414–419.

KÖHLER, W., and WALLACH, H. (1944). Figural after-effects; an investigation of visual processes, *Proc. Amer. phil. Soc.* 88:269–357.

KÖLLNER, H. (1914). Das funktionelle Ueberwiegen der nasalen Netzhauthälfte im gemeinschaftlichen Sehfeld, *Albrecht v. Graefes Arch. Ophthal.* 76:153–164.

KRAINER, L. (1936). Zur Anatomie und Pathologie der Sehbahn und Sehrinde. *Dtsch. Z. Nervenheilk.* 141:177–190.

KRAINER, L., and SUWA, K. (1936). Zur anatomischen Projektion und zur Lehre von der Doppelversorgung der Macula, *Jb. Psychiat. Neurol.* 53:35–44.

KRIEGER, H. P. (1952). Effect of retrochiasmal lesion upon variability of the absolute visual threshold, *Amer. Psychologist* 7:255.

KRIEGER, H. P., and BENDER, M. B. (1949). Dark adaptation in lesions of the optic pathways (abstract), *Fed. Proc.* 8:89.

KRIEGER, H. P., and BENDER, M. B. (1951). Dark adaptation in perimetrically blind fields, *Arch. Ophthal. (Chicago)* 46:625–636.

LANGE, J. (1936). Agnosien und Apraxien. In *Handbuch der Neurologie* (ed. O. Bumke and O. Foerster), 6:807–960.

LASHLEY, K. S. (1930). Basic neural mechanisms in behavior, *Psychol Rev.* 37:1–24.

LASHLEY, K. S. (1939). The mechanism of vision: XVI. The functioning of small remnants of the visual cortex, *J. comp. Neurol.* 70:45–67.

LASHLEY, K. S. (1941). Patterns of cerebral integration indicated by the scotomas of migraine, *Arch. Neurol. Psychiat. (Chicago)* 46:331–339.

LASHLEY, K. S. (1942). The mechanism of vision: XVII. The autonomy of the visual cortex, *J. genet. Psychol.* 60:197–221.

LASHLEY, K. S. (1948). The mechanism of vision: XVIII. Effects of destroying the visual "associative areas" of the monkey, *Genet. Psychol. Monogr.* 37:107–166.

LASHLEY, K. S., and CLARK, G. (1946). The cytoarchitecture of the cerebral cortex of Ateles; a critical examination of architectonic studies, *J. comp. Neurol.* 85:223–305.

LENZ, G. (1921). Zwei Sektionsfälle doppelseitiger Farbenhemianopsie, *Z. ges. Neurol. Psychiat.* 71:135–186.

LENZ, G. (1924). Die Kriegsverletzungen der zerebralen Sehbahn. In *Handbuch der Neurologie* (ed. M. Lewandowsky), 1:668–729. Berlin: Springer.

LENZ, G. (1927). Ergebnisse der Sehsphärenforschung, *Zbl. ges. Ophthal.* 17:1–26.

LHERMITTE, J. J., and AJURIAGUERRA, J. DE. (1942). *Psychopathologie de la vision.* Paris: Masson.

LIEPMANN, H. (1900). Das Krankheitsbild der Apraxie ("motorischen Asymbolie") auf Grund eines Falles von einseitiger Apraxie, *Mschr. Psychiatr. Neurol.* 8:15–44, 102–132, 182–197.

LIEPMANN, H. (1905). Der weitere Krankheitsverlauf bei dem einseitig Apraktischen und der Gehirnbefund auf Grund von Serienschnitten, *Mschr. Psychiat. Neurol.* 17:289–311.

LIEPMANN, H. (1906). Der weitere Krankheitsverlauf bei dem einseitig Apraktischen und der Gehirnbefund auf Grund von Serienschnitten, *Mschr. Psychiat. Neurol.* 19:217–243.

LOEB, J. (1884). Die Sehstörungen nach Verletzung der Grosshirnrinde, *Pflügers Arch. ges. Physiol.* 34:67–172.

MAISON, G. L., SETTLAGE, P., and GRETHER, W. F. (1938). Experimental study of macular representation in the monkey, *Arch. Neurol. Psychiat. (Chicago)* 40:981–984.

MALIS, L. I., LOEVINGER, R., KRUGER, L., and ROSE, J. E. (1957). Production of laminar lesions in the cerebral cortex by heavy ionizing particles, *Science* 126:302–303.

MARIE, P., and CHATELIN, C. (1915). Les troubles visuels dûs aux lésions des voies optiques intra-cérébrales et de la sphère visuelle corticale dans les blessures du crâne par coup de feu, *Rev. neurol.* 28:882–925.

MARIE, P., and CHATELIN, C. (1916a). Scotomes paramaculaires hémianopsiques par lésion occipitale et scotome maculaire par lésion rétinienne unilatérale chez le même blessé, *Rev. neurol.* 29:112–115.

MARIE, P., and CHATELIN, C. (1916b). Les troubles visuels consécutifs aux blessures des voies optiques centrales et de la sphère visuelle corticale; hémianopsies en quadrant supérieur; hémiachromatopsies, *Rev. neurol.* 29:138–140.

MARQUIS, D. G. (1935). Phylogenetic interpretation of the functions of the visual cortex, *Arch. Neurol. Psychiat. (Chicago)* 33:807–815.

MARSHALL, W. H., and TALBOT, S. A. (1942). Recent evidence for neural mechanisms in vision leading to a general theory of sensory acuity, *Biol. Symp.* 7:117–164.

MC GAVIC, J. S. (1947). Visual field defects due to head injury, *Surg. Gynec. Obstet.* 84:823.

MEYER, A. (1907). The connections of the occipital lobes and the present status of the cerebral visual affections, *Trans. Ass. Amer. Phycns.* 22:7–16.

MEYER, A. (1912). The temporal lobe détour of the optic radiations and its importance for the diagnosis of temporal lobe lesions (abstract), *Trans. Amer. neurol. Ass.*, 37th ann. mtg., p. 201.

MILNER, BRENDA (1958). Psychological defects produced by temporal lobe excision, *Res. Publ. Ass. nerv. ment. Dis.* 36:244–257.

MINGAZZINI, G. (1908). Ueber Symptome infolge von Verletzungen des Occipitallappens durch Geschosse, *Neurol. Centralbl. (Lpz.)* 27:1112–1123.

MINKOWSKI, M. (1913). Experimentelle Untersuchungen über die Beziehungen der Grosshirnrinde und der Netzhaut zu den primären optischen Zentren, besonders zum Corpus geniculatum externum, *Arb. hirnanat. Inst. Zürich* 7:255–362.

MISHKIN, M. (1954). Visual discrimination performance following partial ablation of the temporal lobe: II. Ventral surface vs. hippocampus, *J. comp. physiol. Psychol.* 47:187–193.

MISHKIN, M., and HALL, MARTHA (1955). Discrimination along a size continuum following ablation of the inferior temporal convexity in monkeys, *J. comp. physiol. Psychol.* 48:97–101.

MISHKIN, M., and PRIBRAM, K. H. (1954). Visual discrimination performance following partial ablation of the temporal lobe: I. Ventral vs. lateral, *J. comp. physiol. Psychol.* 47:14–20.

MONAKOW, C. VON (1914). *Die Localisation im Grosshirn und der Abbau der Funktion durch korticale Herde.* Wiesbaden: Bergmann.

MONBRUN, A. (1914). *L'hémianopsie en quadrant* (Thèse de Paris). Paris: Steinheil.

MONBRUN, A (1917). Les hémianopsies en quadrant et le centre cortical de la vision, *Presse méd.* 25:607–609.

MONBRUN, A. (1919). Le centre cortical de la vision et les radiations optiques; les hémianopsies de guerre et la projection rétinienne cérébrale, *Arch. Ophtal.* 36:641–670.

MONBRUN, A., and GAUTRAND, G. (1920). Quatre observations d'hémianopsie double, *Arch. Ophtal.* 37:232–238.

MORAX, V., MOREAU, F., and CASTELAIN, F. (1919). Les différents types d'altérations de la vision maculaire dans les lésions traumatiques occipitales, *Ann. Oculist. (Paris)* 156:1–24.

MOREAU, F. (1918). Sur les troubles de la vision maculaire produits par les lésions traumatiques de la région occipitale, *Ann. Oculist. (Paris)* 155:357–385.

MORSIER, G. DE, and BROCCARD, R. (1937). Syndrome pariétal avec mouvements forcés complexes et hallucinations visuelles; contribution a l'étude de l'"automatose" et de la "grande attaque hystérique," *Schweiz. Arch. Neurol. Psychiat.* 40:164–172, 362–371.

MUNK, H. (1881). *Ueber die Funktionen der Grosshirnrinde; gesammelte Mittheilungen aus den Jahren 1877–1880.* Berlin: Hirschwald.

NAUTA, W. J. H. (1950). Ueber die sogenannte terminale Degeneration im Zentralnervensystem und ihre Darstellung durch Silberimprägnation, *Schweiz. Arch. Neurol. Psychiat.* 66:353–376.

NAUTA, W. J. H., and BUCHER, VERENA M. (1954). Efferent connections of the striate cortex in the albino rat, *J. comp. Neurol.* 100:257–286.

NAUTA, W. J. H., and VAN STRAATEN, J. J. (1947). Primary optic centres of the rat; experimental study by "bouton" method, *J. Anat. (Lond.)* 81:127–134.

NIESSL VON MAYENDORF, E. (1907). Ueber den Eintritt der Sehbahn in die Hirnrinde des Menschen, *Neurol. Centralbl. (Lpz.)* 26:786–789.

OPPENHEIM, H. (1885). Ueber eine durch eine klinisch bisher nicht verwerthete Untersuchungsmethode ermittelte Form der Sensibilitätsstörung bei einseitigen Erkrankungen des Grosshirns, *Neurol. Centralbl. (Lpz.)* 4:529–533.

PANIZZA, B. (1855). Osservazioni sul nervo ottico, *Gior. dell'I. R. Ist. Lombardo* 7:237–252.

PASIK, P., PASIK, TAUBA, BATTERSBY, W. S., and BENDER, M. B. (1958a). Target-size and visual form discrimination in monkeys with bitemporal lesions, *Fed. Proc.* 17:122.

PASIK, P., PASIK, TAUBA, BATTERSBY, W. S., and BENDER, M. B. (1958b). Visual and tactual discriminations by macaques with serial temporal and parietal lesions, *J. comp. physiol. Psychol.* 51:427–436.

PATERSON, A., and ZANGWILL, O. L. (1944a). Recovery of spatial orientation in the posttraumatic confusional state, *Brain* 67:54–68.

PATERSON, A., and ZANGWILL, O. L. (1944b). Disorders of visual space perception associated with lesions of the right cerebral hemisphere, *Brain* 67:331–358.

PENFIELD, W. (1954). Temporal lobe epilepsy, *Brit. J. Surg.* 41:337–343.

PENFIELD, W. (1958). Functional localization in temporal and deep sylvian areas, *Res. Publ. Ass. nerv. ment. Dis.* 36:210–226.

PENFIELD, W., EVANS, J. P., and MAC MILLAN, J. A. (1935). Visual pathways in man with particular reference to macular representation, *Arch. Neurol. Psychiat. (Chicago)* 33:816–834.

PFEIFER, R. A. (1925). *Myelogenetisch-anatomische Untersuchungen über den zentralen Abschnitt der Sehleitung* (Monogr. Neurol. Psychiat., no. 43). Berlin: Springer.

PFEIFER, R. A. (1930). Hirnpathologischer Befund in einem Fall von doppelseitiger Hemianopsie mit Makulaaussparung, *J. Psychol. Neurol. (Lpz.)* 40:319–337.

PHILLIPS, G. (1933). Perception of flicker in lesions of the visual pathways, *Brain* 56:464–478.

POLIAK. *See* Polyak.

POLYAK, S. (1932). *The Main Afferent Fiber Systems of the Cerebral Cortex in Primates* (Univ. Calif. Publ. Anat., no. 2). Berkeley, Calif.: Univ. Calif.

POLYAK, S. (1933). A contribution to the cerebral representation of the retina, *J. comp. Neurol.* 57:541–617.

POLYAK, S. (1957). *The Vertebrate Visual System* (ed. H. Klüver). Chicago: Univ. of Chicago Press.

POPPELREUTER, W. (1917). *Die psychischen Schädigungen durch Kopfschuss im Kriege 1914–16; die Störungen der niederen und höheren Sehleistungen durch Verletzungen des Okzipitalhirns,* vol. I. Leipzig: Voss.

PRIBRAM, HELEN, and BARRY, J. (1956). Further behavioral analysis of the parieto-temporo-preoccipital cortex, *J. Neurophysiol.* 19:99–106.

PROBST, M. (1906). Ueber die zentralen Sinnesbahnen und Sinneszentren, *S.-B. Akad. Wiss. Wien (Abt. 3)* 115:103–177.

PUTNAM, T. J. (1926a). Studies on the central visual system: III. The general relationship between the external geniculate body, optic radiation, and visual cortex in man; report of two cases, *Arch. Neurol. Psychiat. (Chicago)* 16:566–596.

PUTNAM, T. J. (1926b). Studies on the central visual connections: IV. The details of the organization of the geniculo-striate system in man, *Arch. Neurol. Psychiat. (Chicago)* 16:683–707.

PUTNAM, T. J., and LIEBMAN, S. (1942). Cortical representation of the macula lutea, with special reference to the theory of bilateral representation, *Arch. Ophthal. (Chicago)* 28:415–443.

REDLICH, E., and BONVICINI, G. (1908). Ueber das Fehlen der Wahrnehmung der eigenen Blindheit bei Hirnkrankheiten, *Jb. Psychiat. Neurol.* 29:1–133.

REDLICH, F. C., and DORSEY, J. F. (1945). Denial of blindness by patients with cerebral disease, *Arch. Neurol. Psychiat. (Chicago)* 53:407–417.

RICH, W. M. (1948). Permanent homonymous quadrantanopia after migraine, *Brit. med. J.* 1:592–594.

RIDDOCH, G. (1917). Dissociation of visual perceptions due to occipital injuries, with special reference to the appreciation of movement, *Brain* 40:15–57.

RIOPELLE, A. J., ALPER, R. G., STRONG, P. N., and ADES, H. W. (1953). Multiple discrimination and patterned string performance of normal and temporal-lobectomized monkeys, *J. comp. physiol. Psychol.* 46:145–149.

RØNNE, H. (1914). Ueber doppelseitige Hemianopsie mit erhaltener Makula, *Klin. Mbl. Augenheilk.* 53:470–487.

RØNNE, H. (1919). Quadrantic hemianopsia and the position of the macular fibers in the occipital visual tract, *Bibl. Læger* 111:215–232.

RØNNE, H. (1936). Die Architektur des corticalen Sehzentrums durch Selbstbeobachtung bei Flimmerscotom beleuchtet, *Acta ophthal. (Kbh.)* 14:341–347.

RUBIN, E. (1915). Synsoplevede Figurer; Studier i psykologisk Analyse. Copenhagen: Gyldendalske Boghandel (German transl.: Visuell wahrgenommene Figuren. Copenhagen: Gyldendalske Boghandel, 1921.)

RUESCH, J. (1944). Dark adaptation, negative after images, tachistoscopic examinations and reaction time in head injuries, *J. Neurosurg.* 1:243–251.

RUSSELL, W. R., and WHITTY, C. W. M. (1955). Studies in traumatic epilepsy: III. Visual fits, *J. Neurol. Neurosurg. Psychiat.* 18:79–96.

SACHS, H. (1895). Das Gehirn des Förster'schen "Rindenblinden," *Arb. psychiat. Klin. Breslau* 2:53–104, 121–122.

SANTIBAÑEZ, G., and PINTO HAMUY, TERESA (1957). Olfactory discrimination deficits in monkeys with temporal lobe ablations, *J. comp. physiol. Psychol.* 50:472–474.

SEMMES, JOSEPHINE (1953). Agnosia in animal and man, *Psychol. Rev.* 60:140–147.

SEMMES, JOSEPHINE, WEINSTEIN, S., GHENT, LILA, and TEUBER, H.-L. (1955). Spatial orientation in man after cerebral injury: I. Analyses by locus of lesion, *J. Psychol.* 39:227–244.

SEMMES, JOSEPHINE, WEINSTEIN, S., GHENT, LILA, and TEUBER, H.-L. (1960). *Somatosensory Changes after Penetrating Brain Wounds in Man.* Cambridge, Mass.: Harvard University Press (Commonwealth Fund publication).

SETTLAGE, P. H. (1939a). The effect of occipital lesions on visually-guided behavior in the monkey: I. Influence of the lesions on final capacities in a variety of problem situations, *J. comp. Psychol.* 27:93–109.

SETTLAGE, P. H. (1939b). The effect of occipital lesions on visually-guided behavior in the monkey: II. Loss and recovery of function as studied by performance on patterned string tests, *J. comp. Psychol.* 27:109–131.

SHOLL, D. A. (1955). The organization of the visual cortex in the cat, *J. Anat. (Lond.)* 89:33–46.

SHOLL, D. A. (1956). *The Organization of the Cerebral Cortex.* London: Methuen, and New York: Wiley.

SPALDING, J. M. K. (1952a). Wounds of the visual pathway: I. The visual radiation, *J. Neurol. Neurosurg. Psychiat.* 15:99–109.

SPALDING, J.M.K. (1952b). Wounds of the visual pathway: II. The striate cortex, *J. Neurol Neurosurg. Psychiat.* 15:169–183.

SPALDING, J. M. K., and ZANGWILL, O. L. (1950). Disturbance of number-form in a case of brain injury, *J. Neurol. Neurosurg. Psychiat.* 13:24–29.

SPERRY, R. W. (1945). The problem of central nervous reorganization after nerve regeneration and muscle transposition; a critical review, *Quart. Rev. Biol.* 20:311–369.

STRATTON, G. M. (1896). Some preliminary experiments on vision without inversion of the retinal image, *Psychol. Rev.* 3:611–617.

STRATTON, G. M. (1897). Vision without inversion of the retinal image, *Psychol. Rev.* 4:341–360, 463–481.

SYMONDS, C. P. (1945). Visuo-sensory aspects on the ocular sequelae of head injuries, *Trans. ophthal. Soc. U. K.* 65:3–19.

SYMONDS, C. P., and MACKENZIE, I. (1957). Bilateral loss of vision from cerebral infarction, *Brain* 80:415–455.

SZILY, A. VON (1918). *Atlas der Kriegsaugenheilkunde, samt begleitendem Text* (Sammlung der kriegsophthalmologischen Beobachtungen und Erfahrungen aus der Universitäts-Augenklinik in Freiburg i. Br.), vol. I. Stuttgart: Enke. See Chap. III: Kriegshemianopsien, pp. 78–132.

TEUBER, H.-L. (1950). Neuropsychology. *Amer. Lecture Series* (no. 81:30–52). Springfield, Ill.: Thomas.

TEUBER, H.-L. (1952). Some observations on the organization of higher functions after penetrating brain injury in man. In *The Biology of Mental Health and Disease* (Milbank Memorial Fund), pp. 259–262. New York: Hoeber.

TEUBER, H.-L. (1955). Physiological psychology, *Ann. Rev. Psychol.* 6:267–296.

TEUBER, H.-L. (1959). Some alterations in behavior after cerebral lesions in man. In *Evolution of Nervous Control*, pp. 157–194. Washington, D.C.: Amer. Assn. for the Advancement of Science.

TEUBER, H.-L. (1960). Perception. Chap. LXV in *Handbook of Physiology*, section 1: *Neurophysiology* (ed. J. Field, H. W. Magoun, and V. E. Hall). Washington, D.C.: Amer. Physiol. Soc., vol. III.

TEUBER, H.-L. *Effects of Brain Injury in Man* (Monograph in preparation).

TEUBER, H.-L., BATTERSBY, W. S., and BENDER, M. B. (1949). Changes in visual searching performance following cerebral lesions (abstract), *Amer. J. Physiol.* 159:592.

TEUBER, H.-L., BATTERSBY, W. S., and BENDER, M. B. (1951). Performance of complex visual tasks after cerebral lesions, *J. nerv. ment. Dis.* 114:413–429.

TEUBER, H.-L., and BENDER, M. B. (1948a). Flicker-perimeter (demonstration), *Trans. Amer. neurol. Ass.*, 73rd mtg., pp. 174–175.

TEUBER, H.-L., and BENDER, M. B. (1948b). Critical flicker frequency in defective fields of vision (abstract), *Fed. Proc.* 7:123–124.

TEUBER, H.-L., and BENDER, M. B. (1948c). Changes in visual perception of flicker, apparent motion, and real motion after cerebral lesions (abstract), *Amer. Psychologist* 3:246–247.

TEUBER, H.-L., and BENDER, M. B. (1949). Alterations in pattern vision following trauma of occipital lobes in man, *J. gen. Psychol.* 40:37–57.

TEUBER, H.-L., and BENDER, M. B. (1950). Perception of apparent movement across acquired scotomata in the visual field (abstract), *Amer. Psychologist* 5:271.

TEUBER, H.-L., and BENDER, M. B. (1951). Neuro-opthalmology; the oculomotor system. Chap. 8 in *Progress in Neurology and Psychiatry* (ed. E. A. Spiegel), vol. VI. New York: Grune & Stratton.

TEUBER, H.-L., and WEINSTEIN, S. (1954). Performance on a formboard-task after penetrating brain injury, *J. Psychol.* 38:177–190.

TEUBER, H.-L., and WEINSTEIN, S. (1956). Ability to discover hidden figures after cerebral lesions, *Arch. Neurol. Psychiat. (Chicago)* 76:369–379.

TRAQUAIR, H. M. (1949). *An Introduction to Clinical Perimetry* (6th ed.). St. Louis: Mosby.

UHTHOFF, W. (1922). Die Verletzungen der zentralen Bahnen und des Sehzentrums bei Schädelschüssen, speziell Hinterhauptschüssen. In *Handb. d. ärztl. Erfahrungen im Weltkriege 1914–18* (ed. O. v. Schjerning), vol. V: *Augenheilkunde* (ed. T. Axenfeld), pp. 303–320. Leipzig: Barth.

ULLRICH, N. (1943). Adaptationsstörungen bei Sehhirnverletzten, *Dtsch. Z. Nervenheilk.* 155:1–31.

VAN BUREN, J. M., and BALDWIN, M. (1958). The architecture of the optic radiation in the temporal lobe of man, *Brain* 81:15–40.

VILLARET, M., and RIVES, M. A. (1915). L'hémianopsie en quadrant, reliquat isolé de certaines blessures crânio-cérébrales; contribution à l'étude des séquelles des traumatismes crâniens de la guerre, *Bull. Soc. méd. Hôp. Paris* 39–40:1234–1237.

VUJIĆ, V., and LEVI, K. (1939). *Die Pathologie der optischen Nachbilder und ihre klinische Verwertung.* Basel: Karger.

WALD, G. (1941). Portable visual adaptometer, *J. opt. Soc. Amer.* 31:235–238.

WALLS, G. L. (1951). *The Problem of Visual Direction* (Amer. Acad. Optom. Monogr., no. 117). Minneapolis, Minn.: Amer. J. Optom. Publ. Assoc.

WALSHE, F. M. R. (1947). On the notion of the "discrete movement"; a critical note, *Brain* 70:93–104.

WALSHE, F. M. R. (1954). The contribution of clinical observation to cerebral physiology (Ferrier Lecture, Dec. 10, 1953), *Proc. roy. Soc. B* 142:208–224.

WEEKS, J. E. (1940). Scintillating scotoma and other subjective visual phenomena, *Amer. J. Ophthal.* 23:513–519.

WEINSTEIN, S., SEMMES, JOSEPHINE, GHENT, LILA, and TEUBER, H.-L. (1956). Spatial orientation in man after cerebral injury: II. Analysis according to concomitant defects, *J. Psychol.* 42:249–263.

WEISKRANTZ, L. (1958). Encephalization and the scotoma. Unpublished manuscript, Psychological Laboratory, Cambridge University.

WEISKRANTZ, L., and MISHKIN, M. (1958). Effects of temporal and frontal cortical lesions on auditory discrimination in monkey, *Brain* 81:406–414.

WERTHEIMER, M. (1912). Experimentelle Studien über das Sehen von Bewegung, *Z. Psychol.* 61:161–265.

WILBRAND, H. (1881). *Ueber Hemianopsie und ihr Verhältnis zur topischen Diagnose der Gehirnkrankheiten.* Berlin: Hirschwald.

WILBRAND, H. (1895). Die Doppelversorgung der Makula lutea und der Förster'sche Fall von doppelseitiger homonymer Hemianopsie, *Arch. Augenheilk.* 31:93–101 (Förster-Festschrift).

WILBRAND, H. (1925–26). Ueber die Bedeutung kleinster homonymhemianopischer Gesichtsfelddefekte, *Z. Augenheilk.* 58:197–201.

WILBRAND, H. (1930). Ueber die wissenschaftliche Bedeutung der Kongruenz und Inkongruenz der Gesichtsfelddefekte, *J. Psychol. Neurol. (Lpz.)* 40:133–146.

WILBRAND, H., and SAENGER, A. (1917). *Die Neurologie des Auges,* vol. VII: *Die Erkrankungen der Sehbahn vom Tractus bis in den Cortex—Die homonyme Hemianopsie nebst ihren Beziehungen zu den anderen cerebralen Herderscheinungen.* Wiesbaden: Bergmann.

WILBRAND, H., and SAENGER, A. (1918). *Die Verletzungen der Sehbahnen des Gehirns mit besonderer Berücksichtigung der Kriegsverletzungen.* Wiesbaden: Bergmann.

WILSON, MARTHA (1957). Effects of circumscribed cortical lesions upon somesthetic and visual discrimination in the monkey, *J. comp. physiol. Psychol.* 50:630–635.

WILSON, W. A., and MISHKIN, M. (1959). Comparison of the effects of inferotemporal and lateral occipital lesions on visually guided behavior in monkeys, *J. comp. physiol. Psychol.* 52:10–17.

WOLPERT, I. (1924). Die Simultanagnosie (Störungen der Gesamtauffassung), *Z. ges. Neurol. Psychiat.* 93:397–415.

ZÁDOR, J. (1930). Meskalinwirkung bei Störungen des optischen Systems, *Z. ges. Neurol. Psychiat.* 127:30–107.

ZANGWILL, O. L. (1951). Discussion on parietal lobe syndromes, *Proc. roy. Soc. Med. (Sec. Neurol.)* 44:343–346.

Subject Index

Author Index

139

Index of Cases